A Gui to Vegan Nutrition

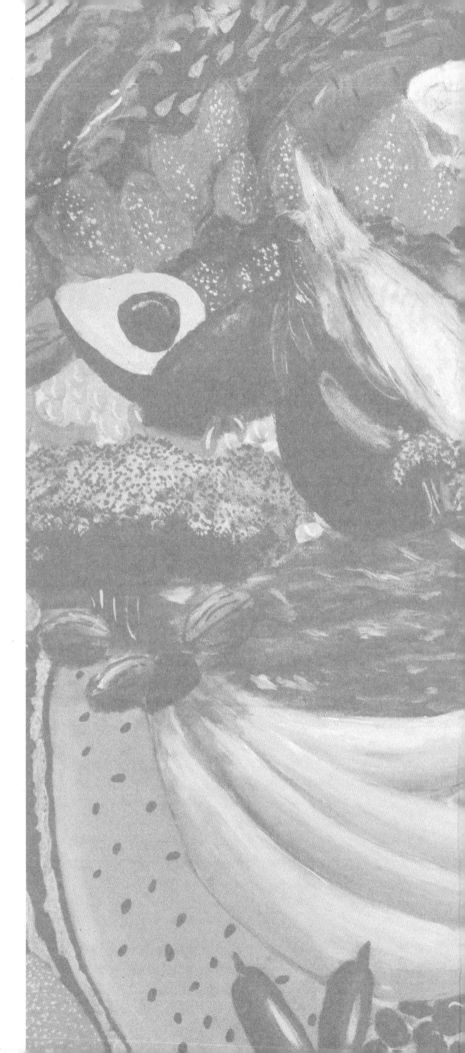

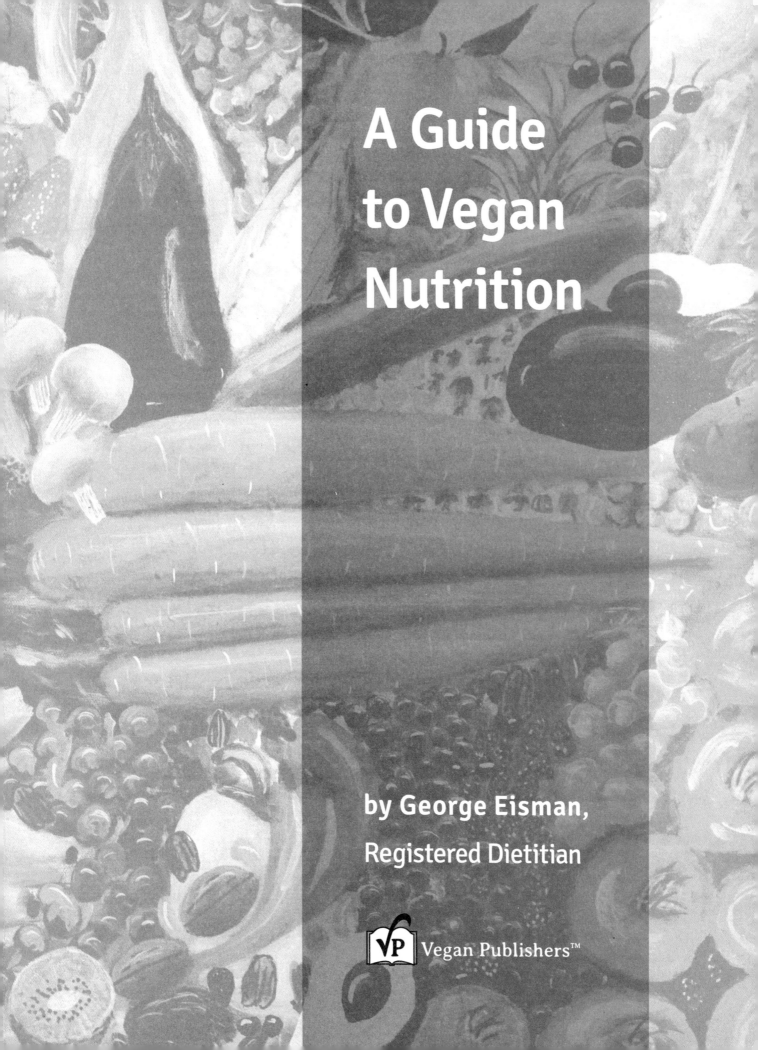

A Guide to Vegan Nutrition

by George Eisman,
Registered Dietitian

Vegan Publishers™

A Guide to Vegan Nutrition
by George Eisman, MA, MS, RD (Registered Dietitian)

Published by:
Vegan Publishers, Danvers, MA
www.veganpublishers.com

Endorsed by:
VEGEDINE — The Association of Vegetarian Dietitians and Nutrition Educators

Sponsored by:
The Vegetarian and Vegan Association, P.O. Box 465 Montour Falls, NY 14865
www.vegetarianandvegan.org

Medical Disclaimer:
This book is not intended to provide personal medical advice, nor does completion of this course qualify one to give such advice under US law.

Cover painting and text illustrations ©Kara Maria Schunk / www.karasart.com
Cover design and text layout ©Robin H. Ridley / www.parfaitstudio.com

 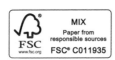

Printed in the United States of America on recycled paper

ISBN 978-1-940184-12-8
Suggested Library Catalog Information:
1. Health 2. Nutrition 3. Diets 4. Vegetarian Nutrition 5. Vegan Nutrition

CONTENTS

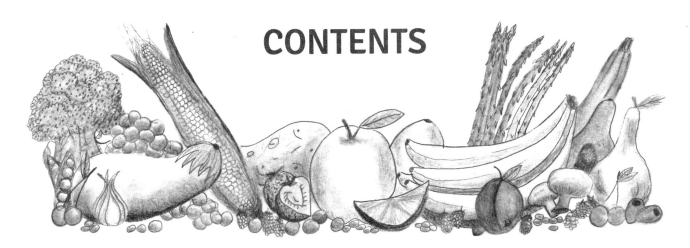

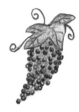

Acknowledgments

Many thanks to my good friend Wayne Cypen for his fine editorial assistance with the original edition of this book. I am also extremely grateful for the encouragement and insightful comments and corrections made by the hundreds of students who have taken this as a course over the past twelve years, acknowledging especially Gail Davis, Terri Reiter, Betty Davis, Gerry Hoffman, Dr. Russ Holt, Dr. Claude Pasquilini, and Dr. James O'Heare. Registered Dietitian Jack Norris, Robert Cohen, and Dr. Michael Greger suggested valuable updates for recent editions.

I continue to be overwhelmingly grateful to the NALITH Foundation of Florida and its founder, the late Jacob Tucker, for their generosity in support of the distribution of this book through the Vegetarian and Vegan Association.

I am grateful to my partner Claire Holzner for her editorial assistance with this most recent edition of the book. Lastly, I acknowledge my mother Rose and my children Sarah and Thomas for their patience and enduring love as I have traveled extensively to speak about this book.

George Eisman
Watkins Glen, New York
April 2015

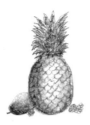

List of Tables & Figures

Preface — About This Book

This book is for anyone seeking basic knowledge about nutrition, but especially for those who are interested in or already following a completely plant-based (vegan) diet. No assumption is made that the reader has any formal training in nutrition. In each unit there are one or more passages marked as "Vegan Point of Information" which specifically highlight information that is unique to vegan situations. Readers who have some training in nutrition science might wish to skim most sections but pay special attention to these passages. The "Vegan Points of Information" contain information and points of view often not covered in standard nutrition textbooks, which tend to overlook the benefits of plant-based diets.

When I first taught Basic Nutrition courses at the college and university level in the early 1980s, I was painfully aware of messages common in textbooks that something was lacking in vegetarian, and especially vegan, diets. I say painfully because I was a vegetarian and aspired to be vegan. I was thus torn between my beliefs and what I was being asked to teach. As the years passed, however, new textbooks, and even new editions of the same textbooks, began to present a very different tone in this regard. Subtle but scientifically grounded passages basically added up to an endorsement of a vegan diet as optimal for the human species.

In 1986 I was fortunate to be hired to develop the United States' first for-credit secular program in Vegetarian Studies at Miami-Dade Community College in Florida. I thus had the opportunity to organize courses based around these types of endorsements, rather than just encouraging students to seek further reference if so interested.

This guide is a compilation of the lecture material I have presented ever since then. It represents the information I hoped students would leave the class with: practical knowledge of appropriate human diets and enough scientific basis to be able to critically read and converse in academic nutrition circles.

As this is a basic guide to vegan nutrition and also a course that can be taken for certification, students should in no way consider themselves nutrition professionals merely by completing it. It should, however, appropriately arm them to at least have a starting point to counter criticism (often by otherwise well-trained nutrition professionals) of vegan diets. The book begins by looking at protein, carbohydrates, and fiber, and then moves on to metabolic factors related to nutrition and considers vitamins and minerals. Following that are two chapters about foods and then two chapters on diet-related chronic diseases. The book concludes with an overview of vegan diets at all stages of the life cycle.

To achieve optimal learning from this guide, it is recommended that the student first read through each unit's **Information Summary** and then answer the questions of the **Practice Test** which is found at the end of each unit. It is suggested that this be done first on a separate sheet of paper, to allow for retaking without bias of previous work. Then the student (or another individual) should evaluate the test using the **Answer Keys**. After waiting a day or two, (s)he should retake the test, continuing to repeat this cycle until a perfect score is achieved.

Enjoy your learning...
George Eisman, Instructor

Introduction to Nutrition

The study of nutrition is the study of how the human body uses food to carry on its life processes. Early nutritionists took a diet-centered approach, looking at a person's or group's total eating pattern and then observing the results in terms of overall health and longevity. Because we have been able to isolate various components of foods and recognize how each is used by our bodies, we now have the tendency to take the nutrient-oriented approach. In this approach, the substances in foods are examined individually, an optimum intake for those substances is estimated, and then dietary recommendations are made, based on which combinations of foods contain the appropriate amounts of those substances. It is certainly a roundabout way of coming to the same conclusions, but it has the pretext of being more precise, and that is of great appeal to the scientist. It should be heartening that science, for all its nearsightedness, eventually leads to the truth.

The focus of this guide is on how the nutrient approach to nutrition can be satisfied using all vegan foods.

The nutrients that human beings need fall into two categories: those that provide fuel for the body (measured in units called calories) and those that are needed for other purposes (non-energy nutrients). The breakdown is shown in the following nutrient chart:

Energy Nutrients	Non-Energy Nutrients
Carbohydrates	Vitamins
Protein	Minerals
Fat	Water
(Alcohol)	(Fiber)

Alcohol is parenthesized because although ethanol ("drinking alcohol") can be used as a fuel source by the body, it is not recommended as a major supplier of energy because of its drug effect. Fiber is parenthesized for a far different reason. Until recently, fiber was not considered a nutrient because it passed through the body undigested. We now know that it serves some very important functions along the way—a good lesson in humility for nutrition scientists of the time. Technically, though, fiber is not an "essential" nutrient (i.e., you will not die from lack of it), but many chronic conditions become much more likely. Nutrition is still far from a perfect science, but in the meantime we all have to eat....

WHY CHOOSE A VEGAN DIET?

A vegetarian diet is one that excludes all meat, fish, and poultry. A vegan diet, as the term will be used in this book, is the type of vegetarian diet that also excludes all other animal products: dairy products, eggs, honey, and anything else of animal origin.

There are many reasons for which one might choose to eat a vegan diet. This section introduces a few of them, while the remainder of this book discusses the ways to assure the nutritional adequacy of a diet and explores some of the health advantages of eating plant based.

COMPASSION

The idea that human beings ought to exercise their compassionate nature in regard to other species is an ancient one. Those who argue that other animals kill weaker animals for food need to be reminded that it is our humanness—our humaneness—that defines modern Western civilization. The notion of being "civil" is the opposite of being savage, where all behavior is based around violence.

When no other choices are available, man has resorted to hunting for survival. When given a choice, it seems the civil one is not to kill. To hold animals captive in order to secure their secretions (milk, eggs) and then to kill them when their productivity declines is certainly not a civil act either. In today's world, obtaining food from the plant kingdom rather than through exploitation of other animal species is not only possible but proven to be very healthful.

ECOLOGY

The balance of nature depends on there being a broad base of plant matter to support the herbivorous animals, who in turn are eaten by the much less numerous carnivorous animals. Human beings have populated the earth to such an extent that choosing a carnivorous diet wreaks havoc on the environment. True carnivorous species are being driven to extinction, native herbivorous species are highly threatened as we fence off their natural grazing lands, and even plant species are decimated as we cut down forests and plant specific crops for our "livestock" to eat. A large percentage of the grain grown in the United States is used for animal feed. The Environmental Protection agency states that "according to the National Corn Growers Association, about eighty percent of all corn grown in the United States is consumed by domestic and overseas livestock, poultry, and fish production."[1] If we all became vegan, nearly all of the crop land used to produce animal feed could revert back to forest and natural grassland, once again purifying the water, soil, and air.

Moreover, the sheer scale of animal agriculture in the 21st century is a huge challenge for the delicate balance of ecosystems and the climate of this planet. As Richard A. Oppenlander writes, "With 70 billion raised each year globally, livestock now consume 45% of the entire landmass on Earth and 77% of all coarse grains grown annually. The land-based animal agriculture industry uses 27% of all freshwater withdrawals, and is one of the leading contributors to climate change, producing between 14.5% and 51% of all human-derived greenhouse gas emissions."[2]

The ultimate in dining in concordance with nature is the gathering of wild edible foods. Though some "foragers" include animal products like shellfish in their cuisine, many books on the subject, like Identifying and *Harvesting Edible and Medicinal Plants* and *The Wild Vegetarian Cookbook* (both by Steve Brill) and *From Crabgrass Muffins to Pine Needle Tea* (by Linda Runyon), are vegan. The latter book, despite its homespun-sounding title, contains detailed nutritional analyses of many wild edible plants. The content of important nutrients like iron, calcium, beta-carotene, and vitamin C is astounding in many cases. Common lawn and garden "weeds" like dandelion, chickweed, common plantain, lamb's quarters, and purslane are as rich as, or are richer in, these nutrients than most, if not all, of the "vegetables" grown in gardens or sold as produce. It seems Mother Nature really wants to nourish us—for free! It is estimated that out of the 300,000 or so species of higher plants in the world, about 80,000 have been found to be edible. Only a small fraction of these are cultivated, making the consumption of wild plants an amazing resource for a truly varied diet. A good way to start becoming knowledgeable about this cuisine is to learn to identify the most common "weeds" that grow in your area; chances are that about one in three will be listed as edible in a wild edibles book such as one of those listed above or in the very richly illustrated *A Field Guide to Edible Wild Plants* by Lee Allen Peterson.

HUMAN HUNGER AROUND THE WORLD

It is estimated that as much as 16 pounds of grain and soybeans are needed to produce one pound of beef. Considering that 16 people could have each eaten one of those pounds, it is certainly extravagant to demand a meat-centered diet when about one-third of the world's children are calorie deficient.

Some argue that the extra grain saved may not reach those who need it, given our complicated and sometimes heartless political and economic system. The truth is that the United States is now a net importer of beef, meaning we bring in more than we send out, depriving hungry countries of 16 pounds of grain with each pound imported. In addition, we set for the rest of the world a bad example of how to eat—not just in that the meat-centered diet is inequitable and will result in a greater disparity between rich and poor, but also in that scarce medical resources will be wasted treating chronic disease.

With rapidly growing human population around the world, consumption of animal products will have to decline dramatically if we are to avoid widespread hunger and famine. In 2012 John Vidal reported in *The Guardian* about research by the Stockholm International Water Institute (SIWI): "Humans derive about 20% of their protein from animal-based products now, but this may need to drop to just 5% to feed the extra 2 billion people expected to be alive by 2050, according to research by some of the world's leading water scientists."[3]

RELIGIOUS (& OTHER) DOCTRINES

Throughout recorded history there have been several religions and schools of philosophy that have recommended vegan and/or vegetarian dietary practices. It is important to have at least a simple understanding of some of these practices, if for no other reason than to be able to relate to individuals in an audience or class who may have strong personal or familial ties with one of them.

HINDUISM & BUDDHISM

By far the largest number of vegetarians (perhaps several hundred million) in the world is in India. Hindus believe strongly in reincarnation, and thus every being has the potential to be, or to have been, a human being in another lifetime. Many Westerners oversimplify this into the "sacred cow" concept (cows are considered a very high level in the reincarnation scheme). Some dietitians have gone so far as to criticize the society for allowing such a "potentially good source of nourishment" for its hungry millions to "go to waste." This is not very diplomatic; it is almost like going into our inner cities and criticizing people for not taking advantage of all the cockroaches and rats they could be eating.

Because of the reverence for the cow, many Hindus put dietary emphasis on dairy products, considering it almost a religious act to share with the calf the nourishment of "mother cow." It is a far cry from the animal abuse in Western dairy industries, so an ironic conflict often arises in North America between vegans and Hindu-motivated vegetarians when the ethical nature of dairy consumption is discussed.

Buddhism is prevalent in various forms in China, Japan, and other parts of East Asia. In many areas, Buddhist monks do not eat meat, and people who are strict in their religious beliefs follow the lead of these holy men and women. A vegan traveler in China recently remarked that he had trouble having his preferences understood in restaurants until he started telling proprietors that he was a strict Buddhist (which wasn't true); they were then more clear about what he wouldn't eat. Many Buddhist-oriented meditation groups in North America recommend a vegan diet as an aid in clearing the mind.

MACROBIOTICS

Taken from the German *makrobiotik* (long life), macrobiotics describes a system of eating that originated in Japan. Its goal is to balance the two extremes in nature called *yin* and *yang*. On one extreme (*yin*) are sweet foods; on the other extreme (*yang*) are meats. Both extremes are preferably completely avoided, or at least avoided in excess. Thus, macrobiotics has come to be considered a vegetarian diet, even though fish is considered less extreme and an "acceptable" macrobiotic diet may include as much as 5% of its weight as fish flesh (though many macrobiotics do not eat any fish at all). What is interesting from a Western perspective is that this balancing winds up advocating a diet with about 80% of its calories as carbohydrate, 10% as fat, and 10% as protein, although it does not use these terms at all.

Another principle of macrobiotics is to eat what is grown locally and in season. However, since the diet was developed in Japan, there are many root vegetables (certain radishes) and seaweeds common there (but not here) that are advocated in food and recipe books. True macrobiotic principles dictate these not be consumed by North Americans, yet these foods have come to be considered "macrobiotic foods." (There is really no such thing: the context in which foods are eaten is all-important, not the foods themselves). So at great expense these imported foods are used in North American macrobiotics, sometimes with negative consequences (besides the expense). Overemphasizing sea vegetables, many of which contain considerable amounts of cobalamin analogues, may have brought on B-12 deficiency in children fed a macrobiotic diet. Macrobiotic adherents also frequently emphasize cooked foods over raw foods, and this may also contribute (by destroying cobalamin-producing microorganisms) to B-12 deficiency.

THE SCHOOL OF NATURAL HYGIENE

In contrast to the emphasis on cooked foods in a macrobiotic diet, Natural Hygiene has a dietary recommendation to eat as much of one's food raw as possible. Originated by Dr. Herbert Shelton and popularized in some of its aspects by Harvey and Marilyn Diamond in their book *Fit for Life*, this way of eating is but one component of a natural lifestyle that includes plenty of sunshine, fresh air, and exercise. Most Natural Hygienists are vegans, though many eat cheese if made from raw milk.

The Natural Hygiene diet advocates simplicity of meals, with just one food or type of food constituting the ideal meal. When combinations of foods are eaten at the same meal, there is a hierarchy of good, fair, and poor combinations that are espoused. This notion of food "combining" (more accurately, food separating) is really the opposite of synergistic concepts like protein combining (wherein different foods containing different mixtures of essential amino acids are eaten together to complement each other's limiting ones). In Natural Hygiene, combining foods is just a begrudged accommodation to people's tastes for variety; it is not advocated for any benefit. The rationale behind this aspect of the diet is to ease the burden on the body's enzyme-making machinery, in the belief that digestion will be more complete if many different enzymes do not have to be made and worked simultaneously. Dr. Shelton probably developed this theory while working with some critically ill patients whom other physicians had given up on. When the body is in a state of illness, especially in wasting diseases like tuberculosis and cancer, the protein-manufacturing mechanisms probably are severely compromised. Thus, enzymes, which are all made of protein, don't get produced as efficiently as they should, and so digestive problems could occur when challenged with a complex meal. For healthy individuals, the benefits of simple eating may not be as noticeable, as a properly functioning digestive tract can produce thousands of different enzymes in a few seconds. The principles of "proper food combining" remain, however, as a cornerstone of the Natural Hygiene way of eating.

SEVENTH-DAY ADVENTIST CHRISTIANITY

This Christian sect follows the teachings of Ellen White, who was a nineteenth-century religious and health writer. She believed the body was a temple, so consumption of unhealthy foods was an act of defilement. Meat was considered one such food, as were several spices judged to be "overstimulating." Alcohol and tobacco were considered improper as well. Thus, the vegetarianism of this group is health motivated through a religious basis. As in most religions, not all adherents follow all its teachings: it is estimated that about half of the Seventh-day Adventist churchgoers are vegetarian, although nearly all refrain from alcohol and tobacco. Studies of this group have shown them to be healthier than the average person in the US, but this was generally ascribed to their avoidance of the latter two drugs, not their vegetarianism.

A landmark study by David Snowden and Roland Phillips on over 50,000 Seventh-day Adventists in California in the 1970s and 1980s proved this was not the whole story.[4] Half of these people ate meat, while the other half were vegetarian. None of them smoked or drank alcohol. The study demonstrated that the meat-eating half was much less healthy than their vegetarian church mates and had a lifespan 10 to 12 years shorter. Furthermore, there was a dose/response relationship between chronic disease and meat consumption, meaning that the more meat eaten, the higher the risk of disease. The study is ongoing, and a significant piece related specifically to diet was published on the *Journal of the American Medical Association Internal Medicine* website.[5]

Many Seventh-day Adventists use meat analogues, which are manufactured from wheat, peanuts, and/or soy to look and taste like various meats. These are used more to gain social acceptance than as a necessary part of the diet, yet many of them are now fortified with vitamins, including B-12, and so are seen as a helpful supplement. Most vegetarian Seventh-day Adventists do drink milk, but there is a growing, even more health-conscious segment, including the prolific authors Agatha and Calvin Thrash—both medical doctors—who recommend and follow a vegan diet. Some of their books include *Eat for Strength*, *Animal Connection*, and *Nutrition for Vegetarians*.

VEGAN POINT OF INFORMATION

Life can be a frustrating experience because of the monumental problems that seem to plague the world at any given moment. With the knowledge that eating plant-based foods rather than animal products can alleviate suffering of both human beings and other animals and reduce the rate of environmental degradation, each of us gains the ability to do some good at every meal. Each dollar we spend on food is an opportunity to send a message about what we want and do not want produced in our name. With the comfort we can receive from this and the good health we will get from eating this way, we can set a joyous, vibrant example others will follow.

NOTES

[1] "Major Crops Grown in the United States," US Environmental Protection Agency, April 11, 2013, http://www.epa.gov/oecaagct/ag101/cropmajor.html.

[2] Richard Oppenlander, "Our Lifeline Revealed Through the Eye of Justice," *Circles of Compassion: Essays Connecting Issues of Justice*, ed. Will Tuttle (Danvers, MA: Vegan Publishers, 2014), 171-181.

[3] John Vidal, "Food shortages could force world into vegetarianism, warn scientists," *The Guardian*, August 26, 2012, http://www.theguardian.com/global-development/2012/aug/26/food-shortages-world-vegetarianism.

[4] Jane E. Brody, "Adventists are Gold Mine for Research on Disease," *The New York Times*, November 11, 1986, http://www.nytimes.com/1986/11/11/science/adventists-are-gold-mine-for-research-on-disease.html?module=Search&mabReward=relbias%3Aw.

[5] Michael J. Orlich et al., "Vegetarian Dietary Patterns and Mortality in Adventist Health Study 2," *Journal of the American Medical Association* 173, no. 13 (2013): 1230-1238, doi:10.1001/jamainternmed.2013.6473.

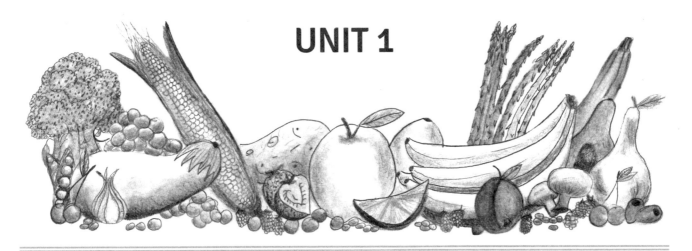

UNIT 1

Protein: Quality

WHY START WITH PROTEIN?

Anyone who has been a vegan for any length of time is probably tired of the question "Where do you get your protein?" The answer to that now ought to be "What do you do to avoid getting too much protein?" Although protein is the building block of most of the substances that human beings (as well as other animals and plants) are made of, it is undesirable to consume too much of it. Indeed, this fact is probably one of the strongest nutritional arguments in favor of a vegan diet. It is ironic that the nutrient most often thought deficient in vegan diets may be the one that brings about their widespread acceptance.

There is no doubt that protein is a vital substance in the body. For example, **enzymes,** the chemicals that catalyze the breakdown of food particles, are all made of protein. Yet enzymes, like all proteins in the body, are built within the body from components obtained from foods previously digested and reassembled. Proteins are not used, or needed, intact. To suggest that we need to eat beef, for instance, in order to build the enzymes necessary to digest it is absurd, or how would we ever digest the very first bite? In short, there is no need for any particular protein: not beef, chicken, milk, egg, or even bean protein. To understand what we do need from protein, a brief foray into chemistry is necessary. (Yes, I know, "Ugh!"—for many of you—but please bear with it; it's not too complicated.)

STRUCTURE OF AMINO ACIDS

Proteins are a class of chemical compounds made up of chains of molecules called **amino acids.** There are approximately 20 different amino acids that the human body uses. Each amino acid is composed of a central carbon (C) atom to which the following four structures are attached:

1. A hydrogen (H) atom
2. An amino group (NH2)
3. An acid group (COOH)
4. A variable side structure

The first three of these are always the same in every amino acid. It is the **variable side structure,** then, that makes the amino acids different from each other. This side structure may be as simple as another single hydrogen atom or it may be a multi-atom complex containing several additional hydrogen, oxygen, carbon, and/or nitrogen atoms. Two amino acids also contain sulfur (S) atoms in their side group (these are referred to as "sulfur-containing amino acids"). What all amino acids (and therefore proteins) do have in common are carbon, hydrogen, and oxygen, which are also the prime constituents of **carbohydrates** and **lipids** (fat) but with the significant addition of nitrogen. Thus, protein can be used for energy (calories) but only after the nitrogen is removed so that it can be burned as a sugar or a fat (the only two substances we can burn for fuel). The significance of this nitrogen removal requirement will become apparent when the problems of too much protein are discussed in the next chapter.

STRUCTURE OF PROTEIN

Proteins in foods are composed of dozens, or even hundreds, of amino acid molecules linked together. Remember that there are only 20 or so different amino acids important to human nutrition, so it is the sequence of them that makes each protein unique. This sequence is referred to as the primary structure of a protein. Think of the English language, in which 26 letters are combined differently to form millions of words. There are millions of different proteins in nature. In the human body alone, there are about 50,000 different proteins.

Proteins also have a **secondary structure,** which is the shape of the chain of amino acids. The chain is usually folded upon itself like a crumpled piece of paper, often with cross linkages holding it in position. Stresses like heat can denature these folds, changing the shape of the protein but changing neither the amino acids nor their sequence.

ESSENTIAL AMINO ACIDS

Of the 20 amino acids considered important to human nutrition, nine are considered essential; that is, they must be provided directly from foods. (The approximately 11 nonessential amino acids can be produced from each other or from the essential ones, if necessary.) For this guide it is not necessary that you memorize the names of the essential ones, but it will be helpful to be able to recognize them. The nine essential amino acids are: **valine, tryptophan, threonine, phenylalanine, methionine, lysine, leucine, isoleucine,** and **histidine.** The human body can synthesize the others as needed, but these nine must be supplied in the diet.

The body's actual need for protein, then, is actually a need for a certain amount of each of these essential amino acids (EAA). A quantity of additional protein-building material, which will be transformed into the nonessential amino acids, is also needed. Invariably, however, when EAA requirements are met, the proteins that contain them amply provide this additional material.

The relative amount of each of these EAAs compared to the amount we need yields a chemical score for any given protein. The EAA that is in shortest supply relative to need is called the limiting amino acid for the protein of that food and thus determines its chemical score.

As an analogy, imagine that you are assigned to make a hundred signs (such as those outside movie theaters that require individual, pre-made letters) that each say "PEACE." You are offered various kits of letters with varying amounts of each letter of the alphabet. Looking at the contents of each kit, you naturally ignore all but the letters *P, E, A,* and *C.* All the other letters of the alphabet are your nonessential amino acids. You require 100 sets of the letters *P, A,* and *C* and 200 copies of the letter *E.* These are your bodily requirements for essential amino acids. If kit #1 has 10 of each letter, then its "limiting amino acid" is the letter *E* (since you need 200 of them). You could only create 50 PEACE signs with this kit, since two *E*s will be used to make each sign. Because your need was 100 signs, the "chemical score" for this kit is 50%. If kit #2 contained 300 of each letter except for C, of which suppose only 80 were supplied, the score for this kit would be 80%. Letter C would then be its limiting amino acid.

Thus, when a food like corn, for example, is found to have a chemical score of 72, it means that if you obtained exactly the amount of total protein that your body required by eating only corn, one of the essential amino acids would be present in sufficient quantity to fulfill only 72% of your need. To obtain 100% of your need, you would have to eat approximately 30% more corn.

The notion of complementing proteins is analogous to buying both kits and combining their strengths to help overcome their respective limitations. Both kits together would result not in just 50 + 80 = 130 signs but actually in a total of 180 signs. The whole would equal greater than the sum of the parts. This works in reality but is generally unnecessary. Frances Moore Lappé's book *Diet for a Small Planet* (1971) popularized the notion of complementing proteins. However, a later edition of that book made clear that it is generally unnecessary, since any single plant protein provides enough of each EAA to meet human needs if eaten in sufficient quantity to meet caloric requirements.

Several facts confound the efforts to accurately assess the "quality" of a food protein. First, there is the constant breakdown and buildup of body protein. Some of the EAAs from broken-down body proteins can be reused to build other proteins. Second, when insufficient calories are eaten relative to the energy requirements of the body, amino acids, including the essential ones, are largely burned for energy rather than used to rebuild body tissues. This situation can make it look like the food protein is of inadequate quality to do its job. This is why it was for so long believed that starving people needed a better protein source when they actually just needed more calories. That's why this condition is now more accurately termed "protein-calorie malnutrition" (PCM). It is protein deficiency induced by a calorie deficiency. Thirdly, there is the matter of digestibility. No matter how good the chemical score of a protein is, if the body cannot break the protein into its component amino acids, it cannot be utilized. Several factors affect digestibility of proteins. Heating a food can affect this positively or negatively by altering the secondary structure of the protein. Tough flesh foods, such as stringy meats, rarely get digested completely in the human digestive system; thus, large particles reach the colon intact. Another factor is the presence of fiber. Recall that an overload of fiber can move digesting food so quickly through the small intestine that nutrients are not absorbed adequately. Protein can be one of those nutrients. In small children especially, a large amount of fiber can result in significant reductions in the amount of amino acids absorbed. Finely chopping or processing foods in a blender helps reduce this effect. (Stone Age people probably prechewed their "baby foods.")

Other measures of protein quality that you may read about, with names like biological value (BV) and protein efficiency ratio (PER), that try to measure how much protein in a food is actually used by a living organism are even more seriously confounded by these kinds of variables.

COMPLETE & INCOMPLETE PROTEINS

One of the persistent myths concerning vegan foods is that their protein is "incomplete," while animal foods are said to contain "complete proteins." The notion that plant proteins are not adequate for human nutrition is an archaic one based on studies conducted on some unfortunate rats. These rodents have much higher protein needs than we primates. The sheer volume of food necessary to meet their protein needs made it difficult for them to achieve adequate protein nutriture on single plant-food proteins. What was (inaccurately) implied was that one or more EAAs were missing from plant-derived proteins and that animal-derived proteins contained them all. In truth, all food proteins contain all the EAAs. The exception is gelatin, which is an animal-derived protein (usually made from the hooves of horses or cows). Gelatin is totally lacking in one essential amino acid (tryptophan), earning it a chemical score of zero. All other food proteins have chemical scores above 30; most common plant proteins are in the range of 55 to 85. Most animal proteins are in the range of 70 to 80. Thus, it is absurd when people speak of vegetable proteins as being incomplete. All that is necessary for any protein (except gelatin) to completely provide for human needs is to be eaten in sufficient quantity so that the limiting EAA is present in an adequate amount. This can invariably be achieved by eating any single vegan food without having to consume excess calories. This is documented in great detail in *The McDougall Plan* by John A. McDougall.[6] The myth of the need to complement plant proteins is thus dispelled.

PROTEIN SOURCES

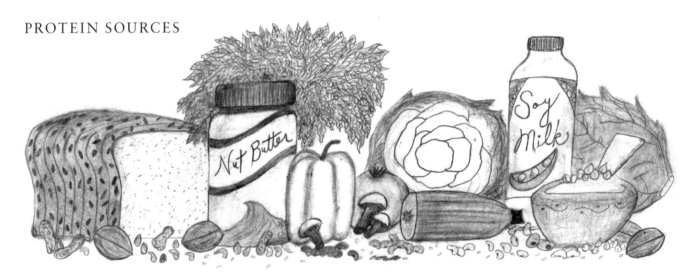

VEGAN POINT OF INFORMATION

If proteins in food are not broken down in the small intestine (the only site from which amino acids are absorbed into the bloodstream), it can be a difficult problem for the lower digestive tract (colon). When this occurs because of fiber pushing everything along too quickly, there is no problem because the same fiber pushes everything out of the colon just as quickly. However, when this occurs as a result of the inability of the body to break down tough animal proteins, bacteria in the large intestine tend to putrefy remaining protein molecules, especially those from meats, and the broken-down products can be highly carcinogenic. Consuming some fiber along with the animal protein helps, but it doesn't make the problem disappear altogether.

SUMMARY

"Protein quality" is an elusive concept in that it is dependent on more than the chemical structure of the protein. It is also a function of variables such as how the food is prepared, what is eaten along with it, and the stage of life of the individual eating it. It is certainly time to bury once and for all the myth that vegan sources of protein are incomplete. Many have chemical scores higher than most animal-derived proteins, and those with lower scores are still highly usable. The high fiber content of unprocessed vegan foods can reduce their protein absorbability somewhat (especially in very small children), but this can easily be overcome by moderately reducing the fiber content. There is certainly no reason to recommend any animal protein to achieve adequate protein intake. Furthermore, with the association between animal protein intake and cancer risk now firmly established, it seems a wiser strategy to get all protein from plant sources.[7]

NOTES

[6] John A. McDougall, *The McDougall Plan* (El Monte, CA: New Win Publishing, 1985) 95-109.

[7] See *Whole: Rethinking the Science of Nutrition* by T. Colin Campbell (Ben Bella Books, 2013).

Practice Test: UNIT 1 — Protein: Quality

Study the **Information Summary** *and then try to complete this test from memory.**

1. The element that protein always contains that distinguishes it from lipids and carbohydrates is:

   a. carbon   b. oxygen   c. nitrogen   d. hydrogen

2. About how many different amino acids, found in food proteins, are important to human nutrition?

   a. 5   b. 20   c. 50   d. 100

3. Of these, how many are considered essential amino acids?

   a. 2   b. 9   c. 17   d. 44

4. What is meant by the "limiting essential amino acid" in a protein?

5. What is meant by the chemical score of a protein?

6. Why is protein quality not determined only by the protein's chemical score?

7. What would you tell someone who tells you he read that plant proteins are "incomplete"?

8. Which of the following is not an essential amino acid?

   a. threonine   b. valine   c. tryptophan   d. gelatin

Answer Keys *begin on page 134.*

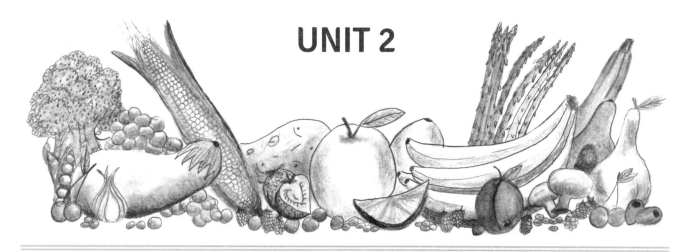

UNIT 2

Protein: Quantity

TOO MUCH PROTEIN?

"Too much protein" is a phrase that didn't appear in nutrition textbooks published before about 1980, and this concept was not given much emphasis until approximately 1990. This explains the skepticism of many health and education professionals because the one nutrition course they may have taken neglected this concept. When too much protein is eaten (more than the amount the body needs for rebuilding and maintenance functions), excess amino acids circulating through the bloodstream are sent to the liver, where the amino group (the one containing nitrogen) is broken off each one in a process called **deamination**. The amino group, once broken off, becomes the chemical **ammonia** (from which the word "amino" comes). This process is necessary because the rest of the amino acid (which now resembles a tiny fragment of fat or sugar, depending upon which amino acid it was originally) is a potential source of calories for the body, which avoids wasting calories. Eating too much protein can make you overweight because excess calories not exercised away turn into fat, regardless of their source. The ammonia piece broken off, however, is where the real trouble starts.

Ammonia (the same substance that we clean windows with) is a very powerful alkali, so to keep liver tissue from being damaged, the body does what you would do if you were washing windows and spilled some ammonia on your skin: it dilutes it. The liver thus engorges itself with fluid (blood) after every high protein meal: a condition known as **hypertrophy**. The liver slowly converts the ammonia into a less powerful compound called **urea**, which is then sent to the kidneys for excretion in the urine. The kidneys are none too happy with this flood of urea, and they too become hypertrophied (enlarged). Engaging in this process meal after meal, year after year, decade after decade, begins to wear on the liver and kidneys (the latter organs more so, because they are more delicate). Kidney failure is a common disease and cause of death in countries where lots of protein is eaten. The condition is rare in countries where poverty prohibits such a "rich" diet. Among populations where a high protein diet is eaten (such as among native populations in arctic and sub-arctic regions) and in subgroups that consume protein heavily (such as bodybuilders), kidney failure is common.

There is also evidence that having excess amino acids floating around in the bloodstream can acidify the blood. The body likes to maintain a blood pH of 7.35, which is slightly alkaline (7.0 is neutral). To alkalize the acid condition, the body dissolves some bone, which is largely made up of calcium phosphate. The phosphate part of that is what is needed as the alkali buffer to offset the acid condition. The calcium is thus broken off from it and is at this stage a waste product to be gotten rid of, since free calcium in the blood will stop the heart if it climbs too high. So, much of that calcium is filtered out through the kidneys to be urinated out. Some is likely deposited in soft tissues, which can lead to hardening and stone formation. Thus, after an acid-forming meal with too much protein, bone material is lost. Doing this over several decades can contribute to the condition of thinned bones called **osteoporosis**. This condition is found in nearly one-third of North Americans over the age of 60, and its incidence there and in other countries reflects excess protein intake much more than it does deficient calcium intake (contrary to what the dairy industry and the calcium supplement industry would like the public to believe).

HOW MUCH IS ENOUGH?

The US Recommended Daily Allowance (RDA) for protein is 0.8 grams per kilogram of ideal (lean) body weight. This refers to the amount of nonfat tissue in a person's body. Since fat is very inactive metabolically, it requires little to maintain itself. Thus, a 200-pound person and a 150-pound person may have the same requirement for protein (and other nutrients as well) if the former carries that extra 50 pounds as fat. "Ideal body weight" is not technically the same as "lean body weight" (because a certain amount of fat tissue is considered desirable and therefore included in the ideal body weight, i.e., added to lean body weight), yet the two terms are often referred to interchangeably in regard to nutrient needs. Both terms seek to discount fat tissue, since it is inert as far as protein needs go.

This recommendation then translates to approximately 44 g/day (grams per day) for the average adult female (120 pounds) and about 56 g/day for the average adult male (154 pounds). These RDAs are based on studies that demonstrated the actual human need for protein to be around 0.3 g/kg lean body weight (translates to 15 to 20 g daily), and then a large margin of "safety" was added to account for population variability. The fact that the average American eats over 100 g/day of protein makes it no surprise that protein deficiency is practically nonexistent here (except among indigent alcoholics). [Metric note: A gram is a unit of weight. There are approximately 30 grams to 1 ounce. A kilogram (1,000 g) equals approximately 2.2 pounds.]

EXTRA PROTEIN FOR BODYBUILDERS?

In the most extreme circumstance of bodybuilding to achieve muscle development, a person increases the daily protein need by a mere 10%. Thus, the approximately 20 g of protein actually needed daily would increase by 2 g to a total of 22 g—NOT a big increase.

LOW-PROTEIN DIETS

When patients are hospitalized for kidney failure they are often put on a "low-protein" diet in order to rest the kidneys. It is acknowledged that the kidneys must work overtime to rid the bloodstream of excess amino acids. These diets are prescribed at 20 to 40 g of protein daily. As you now know, these would be better described as "appropriate protein" diets. No patients become protein deficient at these levels. These diets are, interestingly enough, vegetarian (in fact, vegan, except for the allowance of butter), since all animal flesh is too high in protein to fit into these regimens. It is the only time vegan diets are routinely prescribed, yet they are not labeled as such. It is also interesting that no time limit is set to restrict the duration of the diet for patients because the diet is adequate in every way.

UNDIGESTED PROTEINS

Sometimes protein molecules do not get broken down. Most of these undigested proteins pass into the large intestine (the colon), from which they are eliminated in the feces. If allowed to stay in the colon too long, as happens with animal products that have no fiber to help push them out quickly, they can putrefy and lead to cancer-inducing conditions. In infants, and probably in some adults, some undigested proteins pass into the bloodstream. This is fortunate for the breast-fed infant who can receive the large proteins called **immunoglobulins** in their mother's milk that provide immunity from disease. However, foreign proteins (from foods other than mother's milk) that enter the bloodstream intact are instead likely to cause allergic reactions. This is one reason parents are told not to feed infants anything but breast milk or sterile, easily digested formula for the first few months of life. Allergies are much more likely to develop if foods are started too early before the gaps in the intestine, which allow the large protein molecules to enter the bloodstream, start to close. The fact that older children and adults also suffer food allergy symptoms involving tissues outside the digestive system suggests that these gaps never completely close, or at least can open again occasionally.

It is important to understand the difference between **food intolerances** and **food allergies**. Intolerances, such as lactose intolerance, imply that certain substances in food cannot be broken down normally and wind up lower down in the digestive tract than they should. The result is distress within the digestive system, with symptoms such as stomach cramps, diarrhea, and/or gas formation.

Many people incorrectly refer to their intolerances as "allergies." A true allergy occurs when intact protein molecules enter the bloodstream and trigger an immune system response. (By definition, allergies are always reactions to a protein part of the food.) This may result in such diverse symptoms as skin rashes, headaches, irritability, and/or sinus congestion, to name some of the more common ones. Digestive upset may also be present.

VEGAN POINT OF INFORMATION

In order to lessen the probability of allergic response to natural cow milk protein, milk for infants is heated to the point of protein **denaturation**. This makes it more digestible and therefore *less* likely to be absorbed into the bloodstream intact. The fact that many infants are still unable to drink cow milk formula (whether denatured or not) is indicative of how foreign this substance is to the human digestive system. Many pediatricians now recommend starting infants on a soybean-based formula rather than waiting to see whether an allergy develops.

THE PROTEIN SPARING EFFECT OF CARBOHYDRATE

Proteins are structurally important in all body tissues and also play an important role in fluid and acid-base balance. Their vital role in so many life-sustaining processes is what has probably led to their overemphasis in the diet. However, one use is often overlooked: its provision of calories as an energy source. It is not a good use of protein, but in the absence of sufficient calories from carbohydrates, it is a higher priority use for protein. The body can burn fat for some processes, but others require carbohydrates or protein. In a calorie-deficient situation (starvation, dieting, fasting), the body considers the long list of potential uses of any amino acids available and places energy use (calories) at the top of the list. Thus, a diet with enough protein but too few calories will seem protein deficient to an observer because the protein will not be used for its usual functions (such as muscle maintenance). When conditions are truly severe, even more of the body's proteins (in addition to those routinely broken down but now not replaced) are broken down for energy use. Without fuel, the body cannot do much, therefore fuel is what these otherwise vital proteins are converted into. The presence of adequate carbohydrates (sugars or starches) as a fuel source prevents this conversion. Although fat is loaded with calories, it cannot spare protein easily because there are some human cells, especially certain brain and nerve cells, which require glucose. Glucose can only be made from other carbohydrates or from protein.

FOOD PROCESSING

Protein content itself is not significantly affected by food processing. Heat can *denature* proteins, but this changes only their secondary structure (the shape of the amino acid chain), not the amino acids themselves or their sequence. This may make the proteins less allergenic. Heat, as well as fine chopping (blending, grinding), can soften or break fibers in a food, allowing easier access to, and therefore digestion of, protein.

HOW MUCH IS TOO MUCH?

At least one study has shown that as little as 75 g/day of protein in the diet of healthy young men causes a negative calcium balance (even when calcium intake was much greater than the RDA).[8] This level of protein intake is not much more than the RDA. The phenomenon of hypertrophy of the liver and kidneys is observed when diets exceed 15% of calories from protein. Since a typical intake is 2,000 calories (kcal), this would represent 300 kcal, which translates to, again, 75 g of protein (each gram of protein contains about 4 kcal, so 300 kcal of protein = 300 ÷ 4 = 75 g).

SUMMARY

The risk of excess protein intake far exceeds the risk of a deficiency, especially in this time of reducing fat intake. Most people are replacing high fat foods with high protein foods, when they should be seeking high carbohydrate foods instead.

NOTES

[8] "High Protein Diets and Bone Homeostasis," *Nutrition Reviews* 39, no. 1 (January 1981): 11-13, doi: 10.1111/j.1753-4887.1981.tb06702.x.

Practice Test: UNIT 2 — Protein: Quantity

Study the **Information Summary** *and then try to complete this test from memory.**

1. What is deamination? Why does it occur? Where in the body does it take place?

2. How does consuming excess protein affect the following organ systems?

    a. Liver and kidneys:

    b. Skeletal system:

3. The protein RDA for adults is how many grams per kilogram of ideal body weight?

    a. 0.08   b. 0.8   c. 8.0   d. 80

4. About how many grams per day is the actual human need for protein?

    a. 20   b. 75   c. 100   d. 300

5. How much more protein do bodybuilders require than other adults?

    a. 10%   b. 30%   c. 60%   d. 150%

6. What is meant by "the protein sparing effect of carbohydrates"?

7. What is the difference between lactose intolerance and milk allergy?

8. On a calorie-adequate diet, what percentage of calories from protein is considered an upper limit to avoid risk of liver and kidney hypertrophy?

    a. 5%   b. 15%   c. 30%   d. 60%

*Answer Keys *begin on page 134.*

UNIT 3

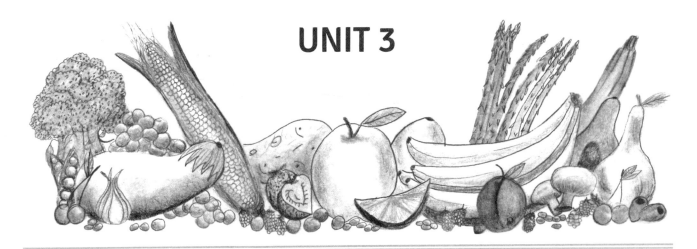

Carbohydrates

Carbohydrates are what we commonly refer to as **sugars** and **starches**. Technically much of the fiber components of food are also carbohydrates, but because they function differently in the body, they will be discussed separately in the next chapter.

As the word suggests, carbohydrate molecules are composed of carbon atoms attached to water molecules (thus hydrated, or watered, carbon). The chemical symbol for carbon is C and for water is H_2O, so carbohydrates are frequently abbreviated as CH_2O or even more simply as CHO. [Note: Most foods are composed of dozens or even hundreds of different chemicals, some of which are nutritionally important (or, more precisely, are presently known to be so). People frequently speak of certain foods in terms of their principal components, such as calling potatoes a "starch" or nuts a "protein." In truth, potatoes also contain a good amount of protein, and nuts have some starch. Both have a considerable number of other constituents. Try to keep from mentally substituting actual foods for components of foods when reading about these components.]

FUNCTION
The function of carbohydrates in human nutrition is as a source of energy. This energy is measured in units called **calories**.

ABOUT CALORIES & KILOCALORIES
In physics a **calorie** is defined as that amount of energy (heat) required to raise the temperature of one cubic centimeter of water one degree Celsius, starting at room temperature. As you might gather, this represents a tiny amount of energy; therefore, in nutrition we take 1,000 of these little calories and call it a "big calorie" or, more accurately, a **kilocalorie**, to measure the potential energy of food and the real energy of the body burning that food for fuel. A slice of bread, for example, has approximately 70 kilocalories ("big calories") of potential energy, abbreviated to 70 kcal. In the popular press, this technicality is generally disregarded and "70 calories" is often written even though, scientifically, that is incorrect.

Remember that foods do not really "contain" calories in the same way they contain actual substances like carbohydrates or protein. Calories only represent the amount of energy that can be obtained from burning the food in our bodies. The amount of calories in the food can only be computed by burning a similar piece of food and measuring the heat output. The assumption is then made that the body will be able to burn it similarly.

Since being overweight is a big problem in our society, it has become the norm to look with disdain on "high calorie" foods. Because the body does little else with carbohydrates than use them as a source of calories, they used to be avoided as merely "empty calories" by dieters. However, in nature carbohydrates come packaged with a host of other important nutrients (the sugars and starches in fruits and vegetables are accompanied by lots of good fiber, vitamins, and minerals, for instance). Yet as commercial food processors removed all this "goodness," not much was left except pure "calories" (such as white sugar). Even in this processed state, carbohydrates rate equally with protein as the least fattening of all the potential energy sources in our food:

Energy Source	Approximate kcal/gram
Carbohydrates	4
Protein	4
Fat	9
Alcohol	7

The above chart contains some of the few numbers from this book that you ought to memorize, along with a good grasp of what they mean. Calories per gram is a measure of energy density, and since excess energy eaten becomes body fat, this represents how fattening a substance is per unit of weight. A balanced diet is one that provides the appropriate number of calories to maintain an individual at an ideal weight. Knowing the above numbers gives one an idea of which energy nutrients to stress in a weight loss diet. There is certainly no reason to avoid carbohydrates, is there?

SIMPLE & COMPLEX CARBOHYDRATES

Carbohydrates are often categorized as **simple** or **complex**. This refers to the size of each CHO molecule in the substance. Generally speaking, what we think of as sugars are considered simple CHO because their individual molecules are much smaller than the molecules of starches and similar compounds (including many fibers) that are thus designated complex CHO. The simplest, or smallest, CHO molecules are called **monosaccharides**, being composed of just one ("mono" = one) ring of six carbon atoms, each with H_2O attached. Thus, they are designated CH_2O_6. This may not seem very simple, but compare them to **disaccharides**, in which each molecule contains two ("di" = two) of these six-carbon rings, or **polysaccharides** ("poly"= many), which usually contain hundreds of these six-carbon rings on each molecule.

The monosaccharides and disaccharides are the **simple carbohydrates**, while polysaccharides are **complex carbohydrates**.

MONOSACCHARIDES, DISACCHARIDES & POLYSACCHARIDES

Here are three examples of each of these subcategories of carbohydrates significant to nutrition (although in chemistry there are many more examples):

Monosaccharides:

1. Glucose—Often referred to as "blood sugar." This is the form that is directly burned in the human body for fuel.

2. Fructose—Often referred to as "fruit sugar." The sweetest of the carbohydrates. Must be converted into glucose in the body before being used as a fuel source.

3. Galactose—A part of milk sugar (see lactose below). Must be converted into glucose in the body before being used as a fuel source.

Disaccharides:

1. Sucrose—Common table, or cane, sugar. Composed of a molecule of glucose attached to a molecule of fructose.

2. Maltose—Principal sugar in grains. Composed of two glucose molecules bonded to each other.

3. Lactose—Milk sugar, found in all mammalian milks (human, cow, horse, etc.). Composed of a molecule of glucose attached to a molecule of galactose.

(A note about enzymes: enzymes are action-specific proteins produced by the body that help break down foods into components small enough to be absorbed into the bloodstream. Disaccharides must be split into their component monosaccharides during digestion, or else they cannot be absorbed into the bloodstream. Thus, sucrose is absorbed as glucose and fructose only after being broken down with the help of the enzyme **sucrase**. Likewise, lactose requires the enzyme **lactase** (which, like all enzymes, is a protein that must be made in the body), or it will remain undigested. About 60% of the adults in the world cannot make sufficient lactase to digest milk properly.)

Polysaccharides:

1. Starch (a part of which is amylose)—The energy storage molecules of most plants.

2. Glycogen—A storage form of carbohydrate in animal (including human) bodies.

3. Cellulose—One of the principal fibers in food.

The enzyme that helps digestion of starch is called **amylase**. It is found in the mouth (salivary amylase) and in the intestine (pancreatic and intestinal amylase).

VEGAN POINT OF INFORMATION

All human infants have the ability to digest lactose (the sugar in all mammalian milks). At birth, infants lack the ability to digest starch. All adults have the ability to digest starch, but more than half of all adults lose the ability to digest lactose. There are no other food components that exhibit this type of pattern. This suggests that milk (preferably human) is the universal staple of human infants, and starch (found exclusively in plant-derived foods such as grains, beans, vegetables, and even fruits) is the staple energy source for adult humans.

HOW MUCH CARBOHYDRATE IS ENOUGH?

Since carbohydrate is not an essential nutrient, there is no such thing as a minimum requirement for it. The amount recommended for consumption each day depends on the total amount of calories needed. As the following chapters will demonstrate, there are definite problems associated with overconsumption of the other energy sources (protein, fats, alcohol), and so it is the limits on these that determine the appropriate amount of carbohydrates. Government guidelines typically recommend that a minimum of 55% of calories should be in carbohydrate form. Less conservative (by virtue of being less influenced by the animal-product food industry) sources indicate that approximately 80% of calories from carbohydrates is ideal.

CALCULATING THE ENERGY NUTRIENT BALANCE OF FOODS

A "balanced" diet is one that derives an appropriate percentage of calories from each of the energy nutrient groups. The typical American diet at present derives approximately 40% of its calories from fat (much too high), approximately 45% from carbohydrates (too low), and approximately 15% from protein (a little too high). Keeping in mind the energy densities of fat, CHO, and protein (9, 4, and 4 kcal/g), you can look at any food label containing a nutritional breakdown and calculate what percentage each of the energy nutrients contributes to its caloric content.

Example:
A food label indicates that it contains 2 g carbohydrate, 2 g protein, and 1 g per serving of fat. How many kcals does a serving contain, and what percentage is contributed by each type of nutrient?

Solution:
2 g CHO @ 4 kcal/g = 8 kcal from CHO
2 g protein @ 4 kcal/g = 8 kcal from protein
1 g fat @ 9 kcal/g = 9 kcal from fat

Now add: 8 + 8 + 9 = 25 kcal per serving

Remember to add kcal, not grams. Now divide each energy nutrient's kcals by total kcals, and then multiply by 100 to get a percentage:

8 ÷ 25 x 100 = 32% of kcals from CHO
8 ÷ 25 x 100 = 32% of kcals from protein
9 ÷ 25 x 100 = 36% of kcals from fat

To check, add the three percentages; they should = 100%.

Practice Test: UNIT 3 — Carbohydrates

Study the **Information Summary** *and then try to complete this test from memory.**

PART I

1–12. Fill in the blanks using the letters of the following choices. Use each choice once and only once.

a. starches	c. cellulose	e. carbon	g. lactose	i. amylose	k. fructose	m. sugars
b. sucrose	d. glycogen	f. maltose	h. lactase	j. galactose	l. glucose	

1. _____ Carbohydrate molecules are composed of these atoms attached to water molecules.

2. _____ Carbohydrates are commonly referred to as these two things (select two letters).

3. _____ Often referred to as "blood sugar." This is the form that is directly burned in the human body for fuel.

4. _____ Often referred to as "fruit sugar." The sweetest of the carbohydrates.

5. _____ A part of milk sugar.

6. _____ Common table, or cane, sugar.

7. _____ Principal sugar in grains. Composed of two glucose molecules bonded to each other.

8. _____ Milk sugar, found in all mammalian milks (human, cow, horse, etc.).

9. _____ About 60% of the adults in the world lack a sufficient amount of this enzyme to digest milk properly.

10. _____ A part of starch; the energy storage molecules of most plants.

11. _____ A storage form of carbohydrate in animal (including human) bodies.

12. _____ One of the principal fibers in food.

13. Why have dieters long been told to avoid carbohydrates?

Practice Test: UNIT 3 — Carbohydrates

PART II

Choose three labeled foods from your pantry (or your neighbor's) and complete the following chart.

	Type of Food	Serving Size	Grams of CHO	Grams of Protein	Grams of Fat
Food 1					
Food 2					
Food 3					

Now Derive the Following:

Note: Do not copy the "calories per serving" from the label. Calculate them from the energy nutrient contributions. However, they should be close to the label number, or you have likely miscalculated somewhere.

Number of calories from:

	CHO	Protein	Fat	Total Calories Per Serving
Food 1				
Food 2				
Food 3				
Totals				
	Total CHO	*Total Protein*	*Total Fat*	*Total of All Three (list above)*

Now—you're going to hate me for this one—calculate the energy nutrient percentages of a meal consisting of one serving of each of the above foods.

Meal 1	*Total kcal:*	*% CHO:*	*% Protein:*	*% Fat:*

Answer Keys begin on page 134.

UNIT 4

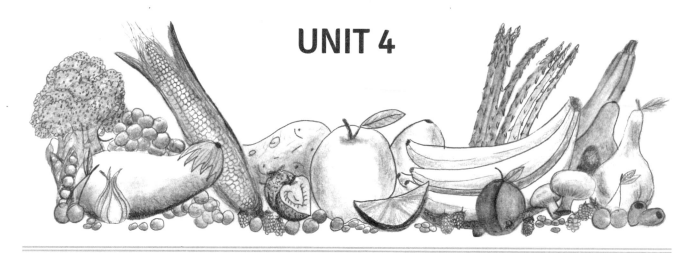

Fiber

Information Summary

In nutrition, **fiber** is defined as the substances in plant foods that are not digested by human digestive enzymes (although they often can be broken down by bacteria). All plants contain fiber to maintain their physical structure. Commercial food processors frequently remove some or all of this fiber to make foods easier to work with or prepare.

Refined carbohydrate is the term used to refer to foods that contain sugars and/or starch but have had most or all of their fiber removed. These may be totally purified carbohydrates such as white sugar or cornstarch, or they may have many other nutrients still remaining. Such is the case with white flour, white rice, or any squeezed (as opposed to whole-fruit-blended) fruit juice. Note that the opposite of refined carbohydrates is not complex carbohydrates, since starch is a complex CHO, yet it may be a principal component of refined CHO. (The opposite of refined CHO is unrefined CHO, which is really just whole-plant foods.)

After perusing the functions (see below) of fiber in the human body, it will be obvious that removing this component from food is not without consequence in terms of chronic disease (diabetes, obesity, bowel diseases, heart disease) risk. The food industry has not been interested in leaving the fiber in food, perhaps because refining makes foods easier to chew, swallow, and overeat (see Function II below). Leaving the fiber in could only reduce sales. Recent publicity about the benefits of fiber has made some commercial food processors grudgingly add a high-fiber alternative to their usual products.

FUNCTIONS OF FIBER
The known functions of fiber are many and complex. Some of the mechanisms have yet to be elucidated. The principal categories of function are:

I. Blood Sugar (Glucose) Regulation: Moderates the release of monosaccharides into the bloodstream to ensure that blood sugar neither rises nor falls sharply.

II. Satiety (Obesity Prevention): Acts like a sponge (most kitchen sponges are actually made of cellulose) in the stomach, drawing water into it, causing a feeling of fullness before excessive calories can be consumed.

III. Bowel Function Regulation (and, not-so-incidentally, Bowel Cancer Prevention): Keeps food material flowing through digestive tract; in doing so helps prevent hemorrhoids, varicose veins, and diverticulosis; also minimizes length of time carcinogenic materials (such as those produced by decaying meat particles) remain in contact with walls of colon.

IV. Blood Cholesterol Regulation: Binds with cholesterol produced by the body to ensure that it leaves with the feces. If this cholesterol is not excreted, it is reabsorbed into the blood; meanwhile, more has been produced, leading to high levels and, therefore, increased cardiovascular disease risk.

TYPES OF FIBER
The three principal types of fiber and their functions:

> A. Insoluble Carbohydrate: Cellulose, hemicellulose
> Functions (see above): I, II, III
>
> B. Soluble (gel-forming): Pectin, gums (e.g., guar gum)
> Functions: II, IV
>
> C. Insoluble Non-Carbohydrate: Lignin
> Functions: III, IV

FOODS CONTAINING EACH TYPE OF FIBER

> Fiber Type A: Fruits, vegetables, legumes, grains, nuts, seeds
> Fiber Type B: Fruits, vegetables, legumes, oats, barley
> Fiber Type C: Grains, seeds, woody (stringy) parts of vegetables

(Rather than try to memorize what is where, it is easier to remember what's *not* where. Note that *wheat*, the staple grain of most affluent countries, is not a source of Fiber Type B. That is what all that publicity surrounding oat bran was all about: *oats* are a grain that does have this type of fiber; therefore its bran fraction is especially rich. The real lesson we should have learned is that eating fiber from a variety of sources is better than depending on one source.)

HOW MUCH FIBER IS ENOUGH? *Daily vs. Per-Meal Recommendations*
After considering what fiber does in the body, it should be obvious that each meal should contain an adequate amount of fiber. It is folly to think that a bowlful of high-fiber cereal in the morning will still be around to regulate one's blood sugar after lunch or to escort the cholesterol out of the body after supper has been digested. Yet most people view nutrition from a "daily intake" stance, so it is common to see "daily fiber recommendations." The current US average intake stands at about 10 g/day, which is definitely too little. Conservative recommendations suggest that it be increased to 20–30 g/day. Assuming three meals daily, the recommendation ought to be 7–10 g per meal. Some reports have stated that at intakes greater than 35 g daily there is blockage of mineral absorption. Other researchers claim that full benefit from fiber is not attained until one eats more than 40 g/day. The controversy will probably endure for some time. (Someone should tell them to stop searching for an appropriate daily intake anyway.)

CALORIE CONTRIBUTION?

Although fiber is not digestible by our enzymes, bacteria in the digestive tract can digest most of the type A and type B fiber. Since these are chemically carbohydrates, they yield about 4 kcal/g. Consuming 25 g of fiber, assuming it is approximately 60% digestible, would yield only approximately 60 kcal, a fairly insignificant amount in a typical diet of 2,000–3,000 kcal. For this reason, fiber is generally ignored as a calorie source.

TOO MUCH FIBER?

Overdosing on fiber is a real possibility, especially if consumed in isolation (removed from its whole-food source). Large amounts of type A or type C fibers can cause too-quick transit through the colon, with the result that many essential minerals might not get absorbed adequately. This does not happen with whole foods unless fiber is concentrated (by eating bran for instance). Small children are much more sensitive to the effects of excess fiber than adults. Consider that the ideal food for infants, human breast milk, has no fiber. This is an indication that the immature digestive tract moves quite well on its own. Adding too much fiber too soon can not only speed things up too much, but the filling effect of fiber can replace more calorie-dense foods and cause total nutritional deficiency. This can happen with whole foods, so it is wise to (at least partially) peel fruits and vegetables and remove hulls from legumes and seeds that are to be consumed by small children under age six.

HOW MUCH FIBER IS IN FOOD?

A typical small serving of fruit (e.g., one small orange, one small apple, one medium peach, or 10 cherries), vegetable (e.g., one small potato, one medium tomato, one-half corn on the cob, or one-third cup sliced carrots), or whole grain (e.g., one-half cup cereal or one slice whole grain bread) contains approximately 2 g of dietary fiber; legumes contain 4 to 8 g per one-half cup serving.

FIBER & FOOD PROCESSING

Processing foods cannot affect fiber content significantly. This can be measured by changes in the glycemic index of the food, a number that reflects how high a person's blood sugar (glucose) rises after eating that food. The higher the blood sugar rises, the less effective the fiber that remains in the food has become. Finely dividing fiber, as happens when grinding whole grains into flour, lessens the fiber's effectiveness: the glycemic index of whole wheat bread is just as high as white bread! Squeezing juice from fruits or vegetables has a similar effect. Whole fruits are much more effective at controlling blood sugar than juices or sauces. This is especially significant because fiber can control diverticular disease. The recommendation for this condition is thus "a diet rich in coarse fiber." It may be that for Function III (above) in general, coarse fiber (usually defined as "no more finely divided than ordinary chewing would achieve") is optimal.

VEGAN POINT OF INFORMATION

There is no fiber in any animal-derived foods. The absurdity by which nutrition professionals have justified not recommending a purely vegan diet is exemplified by the following quote from what was a commonly used college textbook, *Understanding Nutrition*:

It is probably true to say that about 20 to 30 grams of dietary fiber daily is a desirable intake. The diet can supply that amount, given ample choices of whole foods.... However it involves eating such quantities of fruits, vegetables, legumes, and grains that little room is left for meats and dairy products—a way of eating to which some people could find it hard to adjust.[9]

Now, enough said.

NOTES

[9] Eleanor Whitney and Eva May Hamilton, *Understanding Nutrition* (St. Paul, MN: West Publishing, 1987), 79-80.

Practice Test: UNIT 4 — Fiber

Study the **Information Summary** *and then try to complete this test from memory.**

1. What advice (and explanation thereof) would you give to a person who was eating a bowlful of high-fiber (20 grams) cereal each morning and then claimed her fiber intake was covered for the day?

2. Distinguish between simple, complex, refined, and unrefined carbohydrates.

Answer Keys *begin on page 134.*

UNIT 5

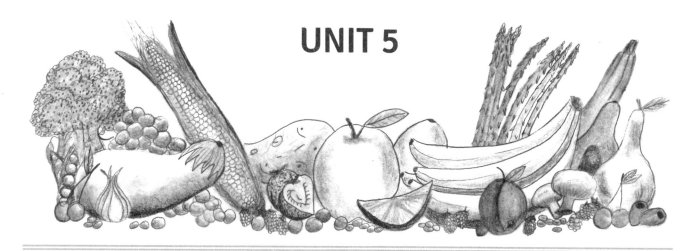

Lipids

Information Summary

Lipids are a class of chemical compounds that include the substances commonly referred to as fats and oils. The three subclasses of lipids relevant to nutrition are:

I. Glycerides
II. Phospholipids
III. Sterols

Glycerides are composed of a backbone of a 3-carbon compound called glycerol, to which is attached one, two, or three fatty acids (chains of 4 to 20 carbon atoms with an acid [COOH] group at the end). Those with just one fatty acid are called **monoglycerides**, those with two fatty acids are **diglycerides**, and those with three are **triglycerides**. Triglycerides are by far the most common type of lipid, both in the human body and in the foods we eat (both vegan and non-vegan). All the glycerides contain just carbon, hydrogen, and oxygen (C, H, O) like carbohydrates.

Phospholipids, as their name suggests, have phosphorus in their structure. The most familiar phospholipid in nutrition is **lecithin**. Lecithin is an important part of cell membranes, and in foods it acts as an emulsifier of other fats. It is not, however, considered an essential nutrient, because it can be made in our bodies from other components.

Sterols are lipids containing just C, H, and O that have a certain ring structure. The most familiar of these compounds is **cholesterol**. Like lecithin, cholesterol is an important compound for carrying out bodily processes, but it is not considered an essential nutrient because it can be made from other compounds. Although some cholesterol in the body is necessary (for instance, it is vital for being able to make vitamin D when sunlight hits the skin), high levels of cholesterol are considered a risk factor for development of fatty deposits in blood vessels (atherosclerosis), which can lead to heart attacks or strokes. Thus, avoiding cholesterol in the diet is looked upon favorably. Since it is not an essential nutrient, none has to be consumed.

SATURATED & UNSATURATED FATS

Each fatty acid can be either **saturated** or **unsaturated**, referring to whether or not it has the maximum amount of hydrogen atoms along its carbon chain. Most glycerides in foods contain mixtures of many different fatty acids, but in most foods one type of fatty acid predominates. Those that are composed of mostly saturated fatty acids tend to be more solid at room temperature; those that are composed mostly of unsaturated fatty acids tend to be liquid. The latter are usually called **oils**; the former are often called solid fats, or sometimes just **fats**. These are colloquial terms, not scientific names. Thus, when one discusses the "saturated fat" content of a food or diet, one is really addressing the amount of saturated fatty acids contained in the triglycerides (and to a much lesser extent, in the monoglycerides, diglycerides, and in some phospholipids).

Unsaturated fatty acids contain one or more double bonds between carbons, instead of having a "full complement" of hydrogen atoms attached to them (as saturated fatty acids do). The unsaturated fatty acids with only one double bond are called **monounsaturated**; those with two or more double bonds are **polyunsaturated**. Most oils and fats contain some saturated, some monounsaturated, and some polyunsaturated fatty acids and thus are referred to as **mixed triglycerides**.

Double bonds are broken apart fairly easily in the presence of oxygen, a process called **oxidation**. This results in a breakdown of the fatty acid into particles called **free radicals**. These now rancid oils have an unpleasant odor, and what is worse is that they are carcinogenic to the human body. Since they have only one double bond, monounsaturated fatty acids have less of a tendency to oxidize than polyunsaturated fatty acids. Thus, the former are considered more healthful in this regard. Although too much of any lipid is undesirable, the current thinking is that the "better" lipids are the ones highest in monounsaturates. Table 5.1 illustrates why olive oil and canola oil are so trendy these days.

Table 5.1 — Fatty Acid Content of Some Oils

Oil	% Monounsaturated Fatty Acids	% Polyunsaturated Fatty Acids	% Saturated Fatty Acids
Olive	77	9	14
Canola	62	31	8
Peanut	48	34	18
Corn	26	61	13
Tuna Fish*	25	37	38

*(for comparative purposes)

Note that while olive oil has the most monounsaturates, canola oil does have the highest total unsaturates (mono- + poly-) and, therefore, the lowest percentage of saturated fat.

Sterols do not contain fatty acids as such, so it is inappropriate to label them either saturated or unsaturated. What is confusing is that the saturated fat content of the diet greatly influences the blood level of cholesterol. The mechanism is not clear, but somehow these saturated fatty acids are involved in keeping excessive amounts of this sterol in the body. What is doubly confusing is that foods that contain a lot of saturated fats also contain a lot of cholesterol (dietary cholesterol), although not always. Some plant-derived lipids, such as coconut oil (and other "tropical oils") contain a high percentage of saturated fatty acids and yet (because they are not animal products) contain no cholesterol. Their saturated fat content does, however, contribute to high blood cholesterol levels. Some fish oils, on the other hand, contain little saturated fat but do contain cholesterol itself. Their total effect on blood cholesterol is minimal. The dietary cholesterol does raise blood cholesterol a little bit, but since triglycerides far exceed the sterols in all foods, the saturated/unsaturated fatty acid ratio is much more influential in affecting blood cholesterol levels.

DO WE NEED TO WORRY ABOUT CHOLESTEROL IN FOODS?

In 2015 the US Dietary Guidelines Committee decided to de-emphasize dietary cholesterol as a subject for concern. This was done because the public had been misled into believing that the amount of cholesterol in a food was the prime determinant of how it will affect their own blood cholesterol levels. We have known for decades that a food's saturated fat, much of which our bodies seem to turn into cholesterol, is much more influential on our blood chemistry than the comparatively tiny amounts of cholesterol already in the food. Consider, for example, that a strip of bacon has only about 10 milligrams of cholesterol but about 2 grams (which is 2,000 milligrams!) of saturated fat. This 2,000 milligrams of saturated fat will turn into much more cholesterol in our bodies than the 10 milligrams of cholesterol already in the bacon. Thus, when foods like margarine and shortening are manufactured they can wind up with a great deal of saturated fat but still have no cholesterol, since they are made from vegetable oils (which have no significant cholesterol content). Producers of these processed foods can proclaim them to be "cholesterol-free," which is quite legal but misleading to the consumer.

FUNCTIONS

Lipids play many important roles in the human body; however, most of them are not essential nutrients because they can be made from other components. The fact that eating an excessive number of calories from any source leads to an accumulation of fat in the body is unhappy proof of this. The only exceptions are what are known as the Essential Fatty Acids (EFA).

ESSENTIAL FATTY ACIDS (EFA)

The two EFAs now recognized are called **linoleic acid** (LA) and **alpha-linolenic acid** (ALNA). A fatty acid called **arachidonic acid** (AA) can be made in the body only from LA, so sometimes it is referred to as an EFA "in the absence of sufficient LA." These EFAs are vital components of cell membranes, so whenever cells break down and need to be replaced (which goes on constantly) there is a need for them.

OMEGA-3 & OMEGA-6 FATTY ACIDS

The location of the double bonds is one way in which different fatty acids are distinguished from each other. One end of the fatty acid's carbon chain is called the **omega** end. Thus, an **omega-3** fatty acid has a double bond in the third carbon position from that end. An **omega-6** fatty acid has its first double bond at the sixth carbon from the omega end.

Much attention is now focused on the ratio between omega-3 and omega-6 fatty acids in the diet because of their roles in blood clotting. The latter tend to promote blood clotting (too much clotting is bad if your arteries are narrowed from cholesterol buildup), while the former inhibit blood clotting (too much inhibiting is bad if you don't want to bleed to death from an injury such as a simple nosebleed). ALNA is an omega-3 fatty acid, whereas LA and AA are omega-6 fatty acids. They can all be gotten from, or made from, the lipids naturally occurring in plant foods.

There are a couple of other important omega-3 fatty acids, namely **EPA (eicosapentaeoic acid)** and **DHA (docosahexaenoic acid)**, that receive a lot of press attention. It seems the human body can make these from ALNA just fine, but flooding the system with cholesterol, saturated fats, or even too much LA retards this process considerably (another argument for a low fat diet). Anyway, EPA and DHA are found particularly in fish oils, so researchers (particularly those who work for companies that sell fish oil supplements) have shown that with a typical high fat diet, fish oil reduces risk of blood clots that can cause heart attacks. This is observed because the EPA and DHA abound in the blood without having to wait for ALNA to be converted into them. On a lower fat diet, the ALNA would get converted more quickly, and additionally there would not be such a need to prevent blood clots if the arteries weren't so clogged up in the first place.

A FOOD ASIDE

If vegans want to boost their ALNA intake (and raise their omega-3 to omega-6 ratio), they can include a couple of tablespoons of flax seeds in their diet each day. These tiny seeds are the richest source of ALNA that we know of; two tablespoons have more of it than a full 4 oz cut of any fish. Be warned, though, that because the seeds are small people tend not to chew them thoroughly. Most of the good stuff can pass through undigested. It is therefore recommended that they be ground up (in a blender or coffee grinder) before sprinkling them on cereal, salads, or whatever. Also, since extended heating can destroy much of the ALNA, at least some of the seeds should be used on cold foods. (Flax seeds blended with water do make an excellent egg substitute in baked goods, but don't depend on these to boost ALNA intake much.)

PURPORTED FUNCTIONS

Other than for EFAs, the other functions of lipids in diet are *said* to be:

I. **Carrying of fat-soluble vitamins**: Four vitamins (A, D, E, and K) are found dissolved in the lipid fraction of foods. The small amount of oil naturally present in carrots, for instance, does this perfectly well; no additional lipid is needed (you don't need to fry your carrots).

II. **Satiety** (pronounced *suh-ty-uh-tee*—"state of feeling satisfied"): Because fats take longer to digest than carbohydrates or protein, they stay in the stomach longer, providing a feeling of fullness for several hours after a meal. (Contrast this with the typical response to Chinese food [mostly carbohydrate]: being hungry again an hour later.) Since fats are so calorie dense (9 kcal/g), there is a price to pay for this satiety. For those who wish to avoid becoming overweight, it is much wiser to seek satiety from fiber, not lipids.

HOW MUCH FAT IS ENOUGH?

It should be clear from the above discussions that the need for lipids is actually the need for essential fatty acids. The US recommendation for these has been set at 3% of calories. Since plant-derived lipids average approximately one-third EFA, this means that a diet containing 9% or more of its calories as fat will meet this recommendation (which in itself is actually very generous compared to minimal needs). For a typical adult diet (about 2,000 total kcals), the equivalent of two teaspoons of corn oil will meet the 3% recommendation. The key word in the previous sentence is "equivalent," since that amount of oil is naturally present in 10 cobs of whole corn (830 kcal) or in 10 slices of whole wheat bread (650 kcal). In fact, it is quite impossible to design a whole-foods vegan diet that wouldn't meet this recommendation. Even fruits and vegetables average greater than 5% of calories from EFA. Yes, we need some fat (lipid) in our diet; no, we don't have to consume it as isolated oil.

CHOLESTEROL SOURCES

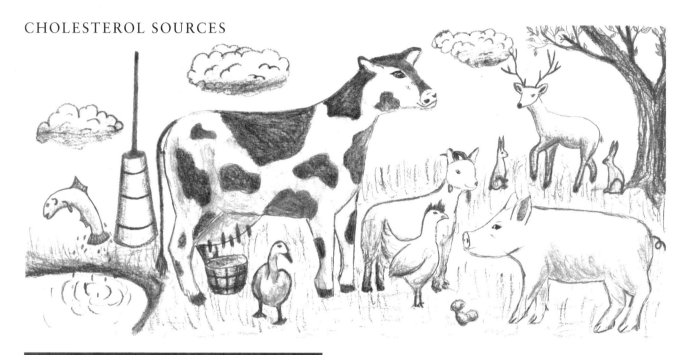

VEGAN POINT OF INFORMATION

Animal fats average less than one-tenth EFA, dairy fat being notoriously low at one-fiftieth. Therefore, just to meet EFA recommendations, someone consuming an all-animal-product diet would have to increase his or her fat intake considerably (to at least 30%). If someone ate nothing but dairy products, she or he could not meet the recommendation at all, since one-fiftieth is equivalent to 2%. No matter how much was eaten, only 2% of calories would be EFA!

CALORIE CONTRIBUTION

The typical omnivorous Western diet derives approximately 45% of its calories as lipids. If two-thirds of this were replaced by an equal weight of carbohydrates, a person consuming 2,000 kcals would not only gain the health benefits of a lower-fat diet but would reduce their calorie intake by greater than 300 kcals per day.

GOOD CHOLESTEROL & BAD CHOLESTEROL? (HDL & LDL)

There is only one form of cholesterol. Cholesterol in foods contributes to elevation of total blood cholesterol. In the bloodstream, cholesterol can be carried by one of several types of structures known as lipoproteins (part lipid, part protein). The lipoproteins that carry cholesterol can be composed of lots of protein compared to lipids, or lots of lipids compared to protein. The former are relatively heavy (dense) because protein is more dense than lipids. (Think of muscle being heavier per cubic inch than fat.) Thus, **high-density lipoproteins (HDL)** are less laden with lipids (including cholesterol) than are **low-density lipoproteins (LDL)**.

It is the LDL, then, ballooned up with lots of lipids, that is more likely to "drop off" some of its load in the arteries, clogging them with a cholesterol-rich material called **atherosclerotic plaque**. Thus, when one's blood cholesterol is analyzed, separate counts are given for HDL-cholesterol and LDL-cholesterol, the "good" and "bad" cholesterol, respectively. It is really all the same cholesterol; it is just being carried differently. A high LDL-cholesterol is considered the biggest risk for artery-clogging disease. Saturated fats in the diet are notorious for raising the LDL count. Unsaturated fats tend to lower LDL and raise HDL. Some worry that it is important to try to keep the HDL count high; however, just aiming for a low total cholesterol (LDL plus HDL) may probably be the best assurance against fat-related artery clogging. A reason for this became evident through some research publicized in early 1993. It showed that there are at least two types of HDL cholesterol. One of them is much more significant in lowering heart disease risk than another. Thus, a low HDL is not bad, as long as most of what is there is this more effective kind. Until blood tests get this refined, it seems most prudent to get everything low.

HOW MUCH LIPID IS IN FOOD?
One of the most important nutrition facts one can know about a food is its lipid (fat) content. Since calories are the limiting factor in one's diet, the percentage of calories as fat has come to be a common measure of assessment. Food labels still, however, usually only tell the fat content (in grams) per serving. This can be misleading when serving sizes are very small, often smaller than what would be commonly eaten. In this way, foods can be labeled "low fat" even though they have a high fat percentage. "Reduced fat" on a food label means that the product has at least one-third less fat than a similar product would. If the original product was very high in fat, this would not ensure that the substitute was indeed low in lipid content.

LIPIDS & FOOD PROCESSING
Cooking does not affect lipid content significantly. High-fat foods can sometimes be cooked in such a way that some of the lipid drains out (such as broiling). In no way, though, can a high-fat food be made into a low-fat food in this manner.

HYDROGENATION
Many food processors add **hydrogenated** fats to their products. What this refers to is vegetable oils that have had hydrogen atoms forced onto their fatty acids such that what once were unsaturated molecules are now saturated. They thus take on similar properties to saturated fats (more solid at room temperature, less prone to oxidation). This is done to create a fatty product similar to butter (margarine) or one similar to lard (shortening). These are added to processed foods to provide longer-lasting crispness in baked goods and to prolong shelf life by delaying the creation of the foul odor of rancid fat. Whether these formerly unsaturated and newly saturated fatty acids contribute to elevated blood cholesterol is a subject of debate. Sometimes oils are just partially hydrogenated, meaning they do not become fully saturated. While this may sound like a reasonable compromise, this process actually creates some unnatural configurations of fatty acids called trans-fatty acids that some studies show are highly carcinogenic.

FATS & CANCER
A high-fat diet has been associated with increased risk of cancer, regardless of the predominating type of fat. The unsaturated fats tend to become rancid, with the broken-down products (free radicals) found to be carcinogenic. When these fats are hydrogenated, as mentioned above, the abnormal trans-fatty acids formed are carcinogenic. Animal fats, laden with cholesterol and saturated fatty acids, cause hormonal boosts related to certain tumors (breast, ovary, prostate). The least harmful middle ground seems to be the

monounsaturated plant oils (particularly olive oil and, to a lesser extent, peanut oil), which are not unsaturated enough to spoil easily yet still are free of trans-fatty acids and cholesterol and are low in saturated fatty acids. They still contain 9 kcal/g, however. There is no evidence to indicate that using them is better or even as good as an overall low-fat diet, especially in an overweight population.

Practice Test: UNIT 5 — Lipids

Study the **Information Summary** *and then try to complete this test from memory.**

1. What are most of the lipids in the human body and in the human diet? (circle one)

    a. polysaccharides   b. sterols   c. triglycerides   d. trisaccharides

2. The only lipids we need in the diet are the essential fatty acids and alpha-linolenic acids. What are essential fatty acids also called?

3. What is erroneous about the statement "Since we need a little bit of fat [lipid] every day to get essential fatty acids, I must add some oil to my salad at dinner each night"?

4. Discuss two other "functions" of lipids in the diet and how they do not justify the above statement either.

    i.

    ii.

5–12. Use the following answers:

    a. saturated fat   b. unsaturated fat   c. both a and b   d. neither a nor b

5. _____ Most animal fats are predominantly this kind of fat.

6. _____ Most vegetable oils are predominantly this kind of fat.

7. _____ Contain about 9 kcal per gram

8. _____ Cholesterol is this kind of fat.

9. _____ Have no calories

10. _____ Increase cancer risk

11. _____ Usually liquid at room temperature

12. _____ Elevates blood LDL cholesterol

13. What is hydrogenation and why is it done?

14. Below are food label statistics from potato chips and pretzels. Compute the percentage of calories from fat for each.

Food	# Calories	Grams of Fat	% Calories From Fat
Potato chips	150	10	
Pretzels	100	1	

15. Cite three dietary indiscretions, two pertaining to lipid intake and one pertaining to fiber intake, that can result in elevated blood cholesterol.

    i.

    ii.

    iii.

16. To which do the terms *HDL-cholesterol* and *LDL-cholesterol* pertain:

    Dietary cholesterol   or   Blood cholesterol?   *(circle one)*

17. What is the difference between *HDL-cholesterol* and *LDL-cholesterol*, and what are the health implications of each?

18. What is meant by omega-3 and omega-6 fatty acids?

Answer Keys begin on page 134.

44

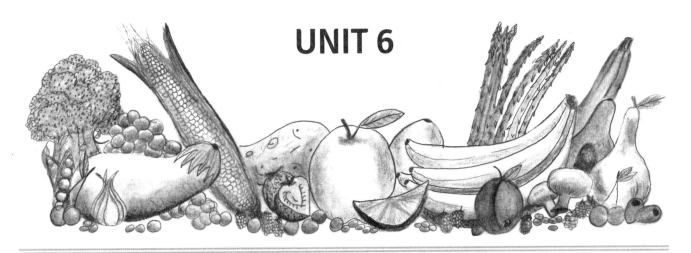

UNIT 6

Digestion & Absorption

Information Summary

This unit reviews the processes by which carbohydrates, lipids, and proteins are broken down in the digestive tract so that they can be absorbed into the body for use. Other nutrients (vitamins, minerals, water) do not require breakdown before absorption.

ANATOMY OF THE HUMAN DIGESTIVE TRACT

Think of the digestive tract as a long tube that winds its way through the upper body, with openings at both ends. The tube itself does not allow everything that enters the mouth to reach the entire body (selective absorption) nor does it allow everything to exit through the anus (selective excretion). Without this type of setup, almost anything accidentally swallowed would kill you, and every time you went to the bathroom you'd risk excreting all your vital body fluids and organs.

The various parts of the digestive system each have roles to play in breaking down nutrients. There are basically two processes at work: *physical* and *chemical*. Physical processes involve breaking particles into smaller particles (of the *same* stuff) and mixing those particles with digestive enzymes. The chemical processes involve these digestive enzymes, reducing the food particles into smaller molecules (making them into *different* stuff).

Mouth: The digestive process begins with biting and then moves to the chewing process. Chewing not only breaks the food into smaller particles but also begins to liquefy it by mixing it with saliva. The saliva contains one enzyme, salivary amylase, which begins the chemical breakdown of starch.

Esophagus: There is a powerful muscle called the diaphragm which lies just under the lungs. The esophagus is a tube that allows the swallowed food to get below the diaphragm and into the stomach. No actual digestive processes go on in the esophagus.

Stomach: While most people think of the stomach as the prime organ of digestion, it really is so only in relation to physical processes. Most of the true chemical digestion takes place below, in the small intestine. The stomach mixes and churns the food material (technically called a bolus when it is swallowed as a solid and then called chyme after the stomach churns it into a liquid). What happens chemically in the stomach mainly involves protein, as the enzyme pepsin begins to break apart some of the long protein chains. The stomach also contains hydrochloric acid at a pH of 2 or less (quite strong).

Small Intestine: It is about 20 feet of coiled tubing that serves as the principal site of digestion and absorption. For anatomy's sake, the first third is referred to as the **duodenum**, the middle third the **jejunum**, and the last third the **ileum**. The total surface area of the interior walls of the small intestine would be large simply owing to its long length, but it is much, much larger (actually nearly half the size of a football field!) because the inner surface is not smooth. The entire length is covered with tiny projections called **villi** (singular: villus), and each villus is covered with tinier projections called **microvilli**. Because of its resemblance to the bristles on a brush, the inner surface of the small intestine is frequently referred to as the **brush border**. It is at this brush border that most absorption of nutrients occurs, since it is within each microvillus that a tiny capillary receives nutrients into the blood from the digestive tract.

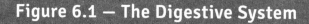

Figure 6.1 — The Digestive System

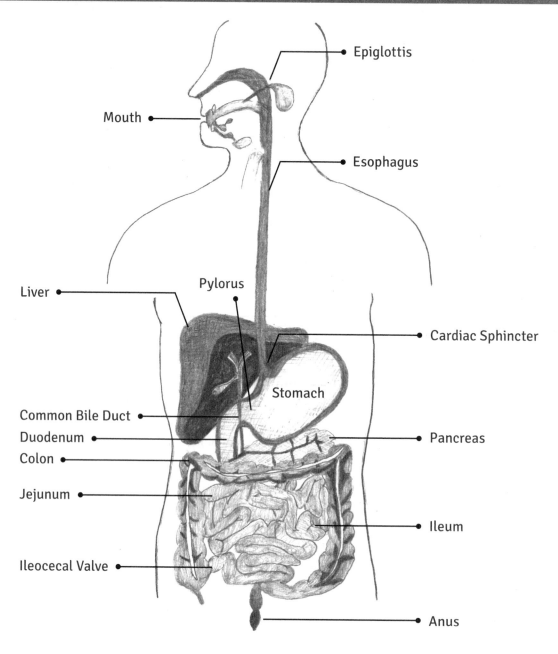

Large Intestine (Colon): The colon is much larger than the small intestine in terms of diameter, but much shorter in length. Its principal function is to reabsorb much of the water (along with many of the minerals that remain dissolved therein) into the bloodstream, leaving a semisolid mass to be excreted as feces through the anus at the end of the colon. Remember that the stomach draws as much as two gallons of water from the bloodstream in order to liquefy foods. If the colon failed to do its job of reabsorbing water, death from dehydration would soon result. During severe bouts of diarrhea, the colon isn't doing this job very well, which is why dehydration is a common cause of death among infants with diarrhea. The usual cause of this, especially in poor countries, is contaminated drinking water.

The Valves: Between each pair of organs there are valves (sphincter muscles) that promote passage of the food material downward and discourage its flow back upward in normal circumstances. Between the mouth and the esophagus is the epiglottis, which permits food to go down the correct pipe rather than the wrong one, the windpipe (trachea). Between the stomach and the esophagus is the cardiac sphincter, so named because it lies near the heart but has nothing to do with it. The pylorus, or pyloric sphincter, separates the stomach from the duodenum. This valve prevents too much of the acidic contents of the stomach from entering the small intestine at one time. This gives the sodium bicarbonate that is injected into the duodenum through the common bile duct a chance to neutralize the acid. Between the end of the small intestine (ileum) and the colon is the ileocecal valve. This prevents the heavy concentration of bacteria in the colon from backing up into the small intestine where it could cause an infection. At the end of the colon is the anal sphincter (anus) which allows us to defecate only when appropriate. We have conscious control only over it and the epiglottis, when we swallow. The other valves work automatically in response to food material in the tract.

DIGESTION OF NUTRIENTS & THEIR ABSORPTION

Most chemical digestion occurs in the small intestine. Any starch remaining (not already broken down by salivary amylase) is reduced to glucose by amylase secreted by the pancreas or the lining of the small intestine itself. All disaccharides are reduced to monosaccharides. (If the person lacks lactase, then lactose remains intact and causes problems lower down in the colon.) The enzymes responsible for carbohydrate breakdown are collectively called **carbohydrases.**

Fats must first be emulsified by a substance called **bile**, which is made in the liver, stored in the gall bladder, and secreted into the duodenum when fats are present. Triglycerides are broken apart into fatty acids and glycerol, although frequently one fatty acid may be left attached to the glycerol and absorbed as a monoglyceride. The enzymes that catalyze fat breakdown are called **lipases.**

Proteins are broken down into their component amino acids. The bond between two amino acids is called a **peptide** bond. Thus, two amino acids bonded is referred to as a dipeptide; three together, a tripeptide; four to ten, an oligopeptide; and more than ten, a polypeptide. The enzymes that split the original proteins are called **proteases**, and those that actually split off individual amino acids are called **peptidases**. To summarize the digestion and absorption of the energy nutrients:

Nutrient	Enzymes Involved	Absorbed As
Carbohydrates	Amylase, Sucrase, Maltase, etc.	Monosaccharides
Proteins	Protease, Peptidases	Amino Acids
Lipids	Lipases	Fatty Acids, Glycerol, Monoglycerides

All carbohydrates are broken into their monosaccharide components before absorption. Thus, starch, which is just composed of glucose units, is absorbed as hundreds of glucose molecules. Sucrose is broken into glucose and fructose (through the action of sucrase) and absorbed as such. Lactose is broken into glucose and galactose (if enough lactase is available) and absorbed. The nonglucose monosaccharides (fructose and galactose) circulate for a while in the blood until the liver gradually converts them into glucose for use as energy. This may seem like an extra step, but for people who tend to have high blood sugar, it is advantageous.

Tiny capillaries of the bloodstream contact the lining of the microvilli of the small intestine to carry the broken-down nutrients (monosaccharides, amino acids, fatty acids, etc.) into the circulation to nourish all the cells of the body. These capillaries carry the blood along with these absorbed nutrients first into the liver, which removes excesses and unwanted materials, and then into the heart.

Some of the larger fat particles, long-chain fatty acids, monoglycerides, and fats like cholesterol (which is absorbed intact) are too big to fit into the capillaries and are instead absorbed through an alternate route: the lymph system. This clear fluid oozes its way directly toward the heart where it is dumped into a large vein, bypassing the liver. This helps explain why dietary excess of fats brings on heart disease, while excess of other nutrients (or contaminants in foods) usually causes liver ailments.

HEARTBURN & ULCERS

The extreme acidity of the secretions of the stomach necessitates it protecting itself with a thick mucus coating over its inner lining. In rare circumstances, this coating does not hold up adequately, and the stomach lining gets burned. This is referred to as a gastric ulcer. Far more common is for this burning to occur just above or just below the stomach itself. Just above the stomach is the cardiac sphincter which connects to the esophagus. The esophagus does not have the benefit of a thick mucus coating to protect itself, so when some stomach acid is let back up through the cardiac sphincter, a burning sensation is felt in the lower end of the esophagus. As mentioned, this area around the cardiac sphincter is close to (but, again, unrelated to) the heart, so this sensation is referred to as heartburn. What causes this to occur? I'm glad I asked...

When too much food is eaten too quickly, especially fatty food (fats take the longest time to digest, followed by protein; carbohydrates are easiest), the stomach expands to capacity and then, not wanting to release inadequately churned-up food down into the small intestine, blows the integrity of the cardiac sphincter to release some of the pressure. Lying down or sitting in a bent-over position immediately after eating can help bring this on. The pain of heartburn is usually such that the individual seeks relief either by discontinuing the overeating activity or by taking antacid medication which helps neutralize some of the acid that edges into the esophagus. It is often mistakenly believed that these antacids neutralize the stomach itself; this is not so. If heartburn is allowed to continue unchecked, there is the possibility of the development of an esophageal ulcer. This is relatively rare, since the pain of heartburn is usually too much to tolerate repeatedly.

By far the most common type of peptic ulcer (the general name given to any ulcer caused by stomach acid) is duodenal ulcer. This occurs at the top of the duodenum, just below the pylorus. The cause is not any malfunction of the valve but rather an excessive amount of stomach acid being present in the chyme, an amount which cannot be adequately neutralized by the sodium bicarbonate (a strong alkali, actually the same chemical as baking soda) produced by the pancreas and secreted into the duodenum. What causes the stomach acid to be so strong? The presence of any food in the stomach causes secretion of acid, but just enough to adequately work on that food. Excessive amounts of acid have been found to be produced in response to these things: alcohol, aspirin, caffeine, black pepper, stress, and meat extract. The first three are self-explanatory. **Stress** is defined as any stimulus that brings about an adrenal response, the adrenal glands being those that produce hormones like epinephrine (formerly called adrenaline). Some refer to this response as the "fight or flight" response (that is, in response to a physical or psychological threat, the mind wants to either fight back or run away). In either event, any food material present in the stomach would become a severe hindrance if it isn't digested quickly. The wisdom of the body is to provide a super flow of stomach acid to speed things up. Doing this repeatedly, however, can cause ulcerative damage to the duodenum.

Why does meat extract (read "blood") cause a similar effect? A long-held theory among vegan proponents has been that the same hormones are produced in the bodies of animals prior to slaughter (consider the stressful conditions under which all animal flesh is rendered, including fish). The animals' bodies respond by secreting a large amount of stomach acid in a vain effort to fight or flee. If even tiny amounts of these hormones are still present in the meat, they could produce the same effect in those who eat it. No other explanation can be found for why meat extract causes the production of excess stomach acid; the scientific community, in its quest for proof, however, prefers still to label it "unexplained." (Perhaps the meat industry does not want anyone to realize the animals it says it prizes so highly are actually ever stressed.)

VEGAN POINTS OF INFORMATION

When asked if small amounts of flesh food are harmful in the diet, many vegans might respond that it is difficult to prove. In regard to ulcers, however, there is evidence that even a tiny amount of meat or fish can cause this oversecretion of stomach acid. Since about 10% of the world's adult population suffers from ulcers, the vast majority of which are duodenal ulcers, it is not a rare occurrence.

In addition, controlled experiments on ulcer sufferers have shown that fiber has a preventive effect on recurrence of their ulcers. Probably the fiber buffers the effect of the acid, not allowing it to make as frequent contact with the intestinal wall. At this stage of your studies you are well aware of which foods contain fiber and which contain none. While it was formerly believed that cow's milk (presumably because of its blandness and "coating" effect) helped relieve ulcers, this is no longer considered valid. Any food in the stomach buffers its lining if acid is secreted in times of stress but does little to help the duodenal lining if fiber is not present.

Practice Test: UNIT 6 — Digestion & Absorption

Study the **Information Summary** *and then try to complete this test from memory.*

1–12. Put the following parts of the digestive tract in their correct order *(the first one is done for you)*:

a. pylorus	d. esophagus	g. duodenum	j. jejunum
b. mouth	e. epiglottis	h. anus	k. ileocecal valve
c. colon	f. cardiac sphincter	i. ileum	l. stomach

1. __b__

2. _____

3. _____

4. _____

5. _____

6. _____

7. _____

8. _____

9. _____

10. _____

11. _____

12. _____

13–17. Match the following food components to the broken-down products they are absorbed as:

a. Glycerol, fatty acids, monoglycerides   d. Fructose
b. Glucose   e. Amino acids
c. Glucose and fructose

13. _____ Protein

14. _____ Triglycerides

15. _____ Starch

16. _____ Sucrose

17. _____ Fructose

Practice Test: UNIT 6 — Digestion & Absorption

18. What is heartburn and how is it caused?

19–22. Select from the following answers.

      a. Amylase   b. Bile   c. Pepsin   d. Sodium Bicarbonate

19. _____ Made in the liver, stored in the gall bladder, and secreted into the duodenum when fats are present.

20. _____ Made in the mouth, the pancreas, and the small intestine.

21. _____ Made in the stomach to begin breakdown of protein.

22. _____ Made in the pancreas and secreted into the duodenum to neutralize stomach acids there.

23. _____ Which of the following does not create excessive stomach acid secretion?

      a. alcohol   b. black pepper   c. caffeine   d. aspirin   e. meat extract   f. fiber

24. Summarize the theory of the relationship between the stress of slaughtered animals and duodenal ulcer risk.

*Answer Keys *begin on page 134.*

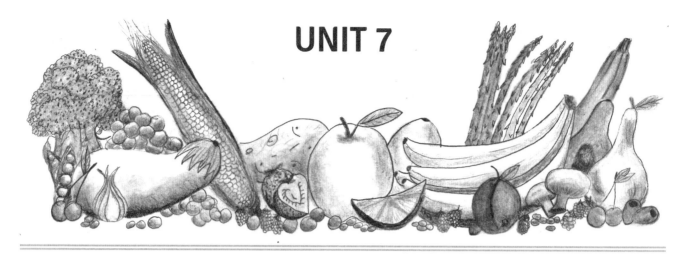

UNIT 7

Weight Control

No single nutrition topic concerns the American public more than weight control. More than a billion dollars are spent each year on weight-loss products. While most people are motivated to lose weight because of aesthetic reasons, there are other concerns. Being overweight increases the likelihood of two serious chronic conditions: hypertension and diabetes. Being underweight does not increase the likelihood of any disease condition, although in its extreme, it leads to starvation. Both situations may, of course, cause psychological discomfort, such that most people prefer to maintain an "ideal" weight. Just what that weight is differs for each individual, although ranges have been set up to approximate ideal weight for any given human height and age. Muscle weighs more than fat per unit of volume, so those with greater musculature ought to weigh more at any given height. What is really sought is a measure of body fat percentage, which is a bit more difficult to derive than simple weight. Thus, body weight is still commonly used to judge this factor. The weight of the human body depends on the balance between calories taken in (eaten and drunk) and calories expended.

CALORIE EXPENDITURE
There are three components of calorie expenditure:

1. Basal Metabolic Energy
2. Voluntary Activity
3. Diet-Induced Thermogenesis

BASAL METABOLISM
The energy needed to carry on the vital life processes, such as heartbeat, breathing (respiration), maintenance of body temperature, etc., is referred to as basal metabolic energy (BME). Contrary to the popular belief that exercise is our principal mode of burning calories, most of the calories an individual burns in a day are to provide for BME. The large amount of energy required was not appreciated until hospitalized patients, who could not eat on their own, started to starve because not enough calories could be supplied intravenously. A maximum of approximately 500 kcal per day can be provided through a patient's arm; this falls far short of an adult's BME needs, even if the person is completely immobile.

The basal metabolic rate (BMR) is approximately 1 kcal/kg of body weight per hour for men and 0.9 kcal/kg per hour for women. (Women generally have a higher body fat percentage than men, and since fat is less metabolically active, their rate is slightly lower.) A kilogram is approximately 2.2 pounds. To convert weight in pounds to kilograms, divide by 2.2.

For instance:

A 150 lb man weighs 150 ÷ 2.2 = 68 kg

His BMR is 1 kcal × 68 = 68 kcal per hour

His BME each day is 68 × 24 hours = 1,632 kcal

Thus, this man burns just greater than 1600 kcal each day even if he never gets out of bed or moves a muscle (voluntarily).

A 120 lb woman weighs 120 ÷ 2.2 = 55 kg

Her BMR is 0.9 × 55 = 49.5 kcal per hour

Her BME each day is 49.5 × 24 hours = 1188 kcal

Hold on! Some people (usually the very diet-conscious) claim they cannot lose weight unless they eat less than 1,000 calories/day. They may be exaggerating, but then again, they may not be. It is possible to change one's BMR by fooling the body into thinking there is a famine going on by starving or dieting. The body responds by temporarily lowering the BMR to conserve energy, allowing it to survive longer on stored fat. When this dieting is done repeatedly over several years, the BMR often becomes stuck at a lower rate. Exercising regularly, and eating normally, generally can unstick the rate. Other factors that temporarily raise the BMR:

Exercise

Pregnancy and lactation

Growth (during childhood, not getting fatter in adulthood)

Fever

Scientists used to believe that BMR decreased with advancing age. It is true that on average a person's BMR decreases by about 5% every decade after age 30. However, it has been found that this is entirely a result of increasing body fat at the expense of more metabolically active lean tissue. Those who exercise regularly, and thereby keep their muscle mass intact, do not suffer any loss of BMR.

VOLUNTARY ACTIVITY

This is what most people think of when burning calories. The difference between what you would burn if you stayed in bed absolutely motionless all day and what you actually burn is your voluntary activity energy (VAE) use. It is actually the sum of the energy required for every movement you make. Physics teaches us that the amount of energy required to move an object is equal to its weight times the distance moved. Thus, if you move your 150-pound body one mile, it would take twice as many calories as a 75-pound child going that same distance. If your arm weighs 15 pounds and you move it six inches, you will use half as much energy as if you had moved your 30-pound leg the same six inches.

The more you weigh, the more effort it requires to move. So on a weight loss program, a 300-pound person can burn twice the calories doing the same exercise as he will burn when his weight is reduced to 150. That is why it becomes more difficult to shed "those last few pounds" everyone wants to lose: more exercise is required to burn the same number of calories. Charts have been developed showing the amount of calories burned doing various activities. These numbers are expressed as kcal burned per unit of time (minute or hour) per unit of body weight (lb or kg). Some examples are given in Table 7.1.

Table 7.1 — Caloric Expenditure of Some Common Activities

Activity	kcal/kg body weight/hr (excludes BMR)
Sitting quietly	0.2
Washing dishes	1
Walking	2
Swimming	3
Bicycling	7
Running	8

A precise measure of VAE would require chronicling how each minute during the day is spent and then multiplying by the appropriate factors. A much easier way to approximate this is to categorize an individual as being sedentary, lightly active, moderately active, or very active and then using the following estimates that have been derived from observing many people over time:

Sedentary (people who sit most of the day, such as office workers)	50% of BME
Lightly active (people who stand most of the day, such as teachers)	60% of BME
Moderately active (people who walk most of the day, such as nurses)	70% of BME
Very active (people who do heavy work, such as roofers)	80% of BME

Notice that these estimates are percentages of BME, because BME takes into account the person's weight, which increases the VAE.

DIETARY THERMOGENESIS

Diet-induced thermogenesis (DIT) is the amount of calories required to digest and absorb foods eaten. [Note: Older nutrition textbooks refer to this as specific dynamic activity (SDA) or specific dynamic effect (SDE).] The average amount of energy required is approximately 10% of the calorie content of the food. Thus, a 500 kcal meal would require approximately 50 kcal to digest and absorb.

This sounds pretty good to the weight-conscious person—almost like getting a discount on everything you buy. Some foods, especially tough proteins, require more energy for digestion than others (although nearly all are in the 6%–10% range). This is one of the reasons that protein is considered more of a "diet food" than carbohydrates. They both have approximately 4 kcal/g, but protein has a bit more of a "discount." It is an insignificant difference, certainly not worth the price of making the body deal with an excess protein load. Loss of appetite, coupled with elimination of refined carbohydrate foods, is what makes high-protein weight-loss diets "work."

A point to consider about diet-induced thermogenesis: where does the energy (calories) come from to digest the food? Even though we say the amount is approximately 10% of the food's calories, those calories cannot come from that food because the food has not been digested and turned into useful calories yet. The energy must come from foods previously eaten, digested, and absorbed. Thus, the first effect of eating is a net drain of energy from the body. No wonder people feel so lethargic after a big meal. Trying to exercise vigorously after eating can result in cramping, as the food cannot be processed properly. Now you know why you were told not to swim until an hour after eating, and why it is wise to "starve a fever" (to not drain energy the body needs to keep its temperature high enough to fight infection).

GAINING & LOSING BODY FAT

Excess intake of calories over expenditure leads to a gain in body weight. Other than in periods of growth (childhood, pregnancy, lactation, bodybuilding) this results in storage of body fat. One pound of body fat (adipose tissue) represents storage of 3,500 kcal. To lose this pound of body fat requires expending 3,500 kcal more than is being eaten.

For those of you who are mathematically inclined, you might observe that a pound of pure fat, which converts to 454 grams, ought to contain 454 × 9 kcal/g = 4,086 kcal. Since adipose tissue does contain some water and protein, the total is lowered to 3,500 kcal. If an individual eats 500 kcal a day more than she burns off, there will be a slight gain of weight, resulting in an additional pound of fat every 3,500 ÷ 500 = 7 days. On the other hand, if she eats 350 kcal less that she burns each day, she can expect to lose fat at a rate of one pound every 3,500 ÷ 350 = 10 days.

Since most average-sized, normally active adults burn between 2,000 and 3,000 kcal daily, it is virtually impossible to lose as much as a pound of fat a day, even if nothing is eaten. Crash diets that advertise loss of anything like that are referring not to fat loss but to larger losses of water and some protein that are both quickly regained once one eats normally again. True fat loss can only be done slowly, and for most people this is best done at the rate of 1 to 2 lbs/week. This represents calorie deficits of 500–1,000 kcal per day.

TOTAL ENERGY EXPENDITURE

Combining the three factors above, total energy use and weight balance can be approximated.

Example:
A 220-pound man is moderately active and eats 3,000 kcal daily. How many kcals does he burn each day? Will he be gaining or losing weight on his present diet? How quickly is he gaining or losing fat?

Solution:
220 lbs = 220 ÷ 2.2 kg = 100 kg
BME = 1 kcal/kg/hr × 24 hours × 100 kg = 2,400 kcal
VAE = 70% × 2,400 = 1,680 kcal
DIT = 3,000 kcal × 10% = 300 kcal
Total burned = 2,400 + 1,680 + 300 = 4,380 kcal
4,380 is more than the 3,000 he is eating; therefore, he would be losing weight.
Daily kcal deficit = 4,380 - 3,000 = **1,380 kcal**
Therefore, he will shed a pound of fat (3,500 kcal) every:
3,500 ÷ 1,380 = 2.5 days

WEIGHT LOSS PRODUCTS

Traditionally, weight loss products fall into two categories:

1. Those that suppress appetite
2. Those that replace more calorie-dense foods

Although those in the first category are generally drugs and fall out of the scope of a nutrition guide, suffice it to say that not only are these drugs often addicting and/or laden with adverse side effects, but they also do not work in the long run. When appetite is allowed to return to normal, overeating usually results in order to restore the body to its original size. Those in the second category are interesting to the nutritionist, if only for the types of foods they seek to replace. The most well-known subgroup in this category is artificial sweeteners. These were originally developed for use by diabetic patients who had to strictly monitor their simple carbohydrate intake. These sweeteners could be used freely so that the individuals could "treat" themselves without calculation. These sweeteners are now much more frequently used by those who are overweight, although their intent has not changed. Note in the statement on foods containing artificial sweeteners that they are meant for those "who must limit their intake of ordinary sweets." Many misinterpret this to mean anybody who is overweight, but as you know by now the calorie content of sugar is not high. Furthermore, it has been shown that the natural craving we have for sweets is not thwarted by these chemical replacements, and the use of them does not result in weight loss. It has been found that the 20 kcal not used as a spoonful of sugar in coffee or tea is made up for by an extra bite of sandwich or dessert.

As far as safety is concerned, the two most commonly used artificial sweeteners before the 1980s, saccharin and cyclamate, were banned in Canada and the United States. Now aspartame (marketed as NutraSweet) has captured the market, although its safety continues to be questioned. A new approach to replacing calories is the development of artificial fats (such as "Simplesse"). There is probably no real craving for fat itself, so this may prove more effective (but perhaps no more safe). In addition, replacing 9 kcal/g does a lot more than replacing 4 kcal/g. Another approach that has been used for a long time is the fiber supplement. This involves taking some form of concentrated fiber before meals to bring on a feeling of fullness. Usually this is in a candy or tablet form, but it would obviously make much more sense to just consume some whole vegetables and/or fruits before eating. How about a fresh fruit cup and then a big salad as the first two (or the only two) courses of a meal? Quite a novel idea, isn't it?

Practice Test: UNIT 7 — Weight Control

Study the **Information Summary** *and then try to complete this test from memory.**

1. The basal metabolic rate (BMR) for normal adult men is 1.0 kcal per kg body weight per what unit of time?

    a. second   b. minute   c. hour   d. week

2. Do adult women have a slightly lower or higher BMR than men?

3. Place an "R" next to the following conditions that raise the BMR and an "L" next to those that lower the BMR.

    _____ Childhood (Growth)

    _____ Pregnancy

    _____ Starvation

    _____ Strict dieting

    _____ Fasting

    _____ Fever

    _____ Lactation

4. Mr. A burns 2,000 kcal daily just for basal metabolism. He leads a sedentary lifestyle. How many additional kcals does he probably burn for voluntary activities?

    a. 10   b. 100   c. 1,000   d. 10,000

5. If Mr. A changed to a lightly active lifestyle, how many more kcals would he then burn each day?

    a. 20   b. 200   c. 2,000   d. 20,000

6. After eating a typical heavy supper of 900 kcals, Mrs. B says she feels very tired. How many kcals is she expending just digesting and absorbing this meal (diet-induced thermogenesis)?

    a. 9   b. 19   c. 39   d. 90

7. How many kcals does one pound of body fat represent?

    a. 35   b. 350   c. 3,500   d. 35,000

 57

Practice Test: UNIT 7 — Weight Control

8. If someone eats just enough to keep their weight stable but one day decides to eat a 175 kcal candy bar after lunch every day, how many days will it be before one pound of body fat is gained?

   a. 2   b. 20   c. 200   d. 350

   How many pounds will be gained at the end of one year?

Putting It All Together

9. A woman weighs 110 pounds (50 kg) and is very active. She plans to eat a 2,000 kcal diet. Will she gain or lose weight, and how quickly will a pound of fat be gained or lost?

   _____ = BME

   _____ = VAE

   _____ = DIT

   _____ = total calorie expenditure

   _____ kcal daily = rate of gain or loss *(circle one)* of fat

   _____ = number of days to gain or lose *(circle one)* a pound of fat

Answer Keys begin on page 134.

UNIT 8

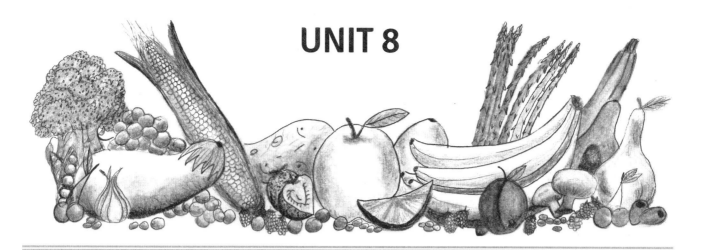

Fat-Soluble Vitamins

OVERVIEW OF VITAMINS & MINERALS

The next several chapters deal with what are called **micronutrients**, in that they are generally consumed in very small amounts compared to carbohydrates, lipids, and protein. They are no less important, because deficiencies of micronutrients can cause serious disease and ultimately death. They are, however, much more prone to be processed into pill form as supplements because of the small amounts required. Nature does provide them amply in whole fresh foods, and that is certainly the preferred way to consume them. One problem with pills is that knowledge of nutrition is incomplete; much guesswork is involved. In addition, there are interactions between micronutrients, such that taking too much of one may crowd out others from being absorbed. Some of these "others" that get crowded out may be as yet undiscovered.

The difference between vitamins and minerals is that the former are organic molecules, while the latter are inorganic substances. This is in the chemist's sense of the word "organic," not in the agricultural sense. Chemically, organic molecules are technically those that contain carbon atoms in certain configurations, with the implication being that they came from living organisms. Minerals are part of rocks; they were never alive. Although chemists can now synthesize organic molecules from inorganic materials, one could still argue that the chemists are the living organisms making them.

From a nutritionist's standpoint, the difference is relevant: vitamins, like living beings, are subject to breakdown over time, whereas minerals never change. Thus, one should rightly be concerned about loss of vitamins during food preparation and storage, whereas minerals are either in the food from the start or not and can only be lost by removing part of the food.

OVERVIEW OF VITAMINS

Vitamins are organic essential nutrients needed in minute amounts by human beings. There are presently thirteen vitamins recognized in the United States. These are generally divided into two categories: the fat-soluble vitamins (A, D, E, and K) and the water-soluble vitamins (Bs and C). The distinction is made not only to point out where to find them chemically in foods (lipid fraction or watery fraction), but also to demonstrate how they are handled in the body. Since fats are calorie-containing nutrients, the body tends to hold on to them. Water is excreted freely, along with anything carried by it. Therefore, fat-soluble vitamins are generally stored in the body for longer periods of time (more than a day). Water-soluble vitamins that are not immediately needed are flushed out in the urine and thus must be consumed more frequently. The notable exception is vitamin B-12, which, although being water-soluble, is stored in amounts that can last three to five years. The flip side of the storage issue with fat- vs. water-soluble vitamins is that there is much more danger of damage from overdose of the fat-soluble ones.

VITAMIN A

Best known for its role in vision, vitamin A also has several other functions in the body, one of the most notable of which has to do with bone growth. When bones grow, they must first be broken down a bit, then stretched, and then rebuilt. Vitamin A is necessary for the first step to occur—the breaking-down process. As you might expect, children deprived of vitamin A do not grow very well.

As regards vision, vitamin A does not improve eyesight that is faulty due to far- or near-sightedness or such diseases as glaucoma. What it does do is optimize night vision, the ability to recover vision after being assaulted with bright light in a darkened situation. So if you are driving at night and it takes you more than a few seconds to see well after an oncoming car's headlights flashed in your eyes, you may benefit from some additional vitamin A. No amount of it will allow you to see as well as a cat does, however. As with all nutrients, you need what you need; you don't need more than you need. Because something corrects a symptom of its deficiency does not imply that a larger dose will provide a super benefit.

Vitamin A also has antioxidant properties, meaning that it combines readily with oxygen. The other two vitamins that function as antioxidants are vitamin E and vitamin C. Since the amount of C and E in foods far exceeds that of A, they act to spare the latter from being inactivated by oxygen. Vitamin A exists in two basic forms in foods. One is **beta-carotene**, a yellow-orange pigment found widely in the plant kingdom. The other is called pre-formed vitamin A, the most common form of which is **retinol**. Pre-formed vitamin A is only found in animal products. The human body can easily transform beta-carotene into vitamin A as needed. When the body has made sufficient vitamin A, the beta-carotene is left to circulate and then is slowly excreted. The only effect of overdose is a harmless orange cast to the skin. However, overdoses of pre-formed vitamin A can be serious. Most of the ingested excess of pre-formed A is stored in the liver, and too much of it can cause liver damage. Some of it gets to the bones, where it does its job of dissolving bone material too well, contributing to development of osteoporosis.

VEGAN POINT OF INFORMATION

Beta-carotene is only obtained from plant sources. Pre-formed vitamin A is only found in animal products or supplements derived from them. This is one of the most compelling arguments for looking to vegan foods for adequate yet safe sources of nutrients. The content of vitamin A in foods is now usually stated as retinol equivalents (RE), although some older tables may still use international units (IU). RE is used more now because it reflects the fact that approximately six units of beta-carotene are converted to one unit of retinol. The RDA of 1,000 RE can still easily be met with half a carrot (1,012 RE), half a sweet potato (1,244 RE), or two-thirds of a cantaloupe (1,290 RE). Again, exceeding the RDA from these plant sources is harmless. Retinol equivalence merely implies how much retinol could be made, if the body needs it.

VITAMIN D

Vitamin D, also known as calciferol, is actually a hormone necessary for absorption of calcium into the blood, both from food material in the intestine and from our own bones. There is a strong argument about whether vitamin D should be classed as a vitamin at all. With adequate sun exposure (generally about five minutes a day, three times a week, face and arms) the human body can make all that it needs. However, several decades ago, many children were kept indoors or covered head to toe with clothing and for that reason could not manufacture enough. Since vitamin D is necessary for proper bone growth, children actually need more of it than adults, who are already fully grown. The child's RDA for vitamin D is actually twice that recommended for adults.

A deficiency of vitamin D causes inadequate mineralization of bone, since not enough calcium is made available to build it as rigidly as it should be. In children, this is known as rickets and results in bowleggedness when the child stands up, as the weight of the body causes the soft bones to bend out. One must be careful in correcting this condition, since if it is done with diet alone the bones may permanently harden in that position. Orthopedic braces are usually necessary to support the legs in a straight position while the bones grow harder.

In adults, this deficiency condition (as is a calcium deficiency) is called osteomalacia. This literally means "soft bones" and is different from osteoporosis, "porous bones." Osteomalacia, much rarer than osteoporosis, is characterized by bones that bend on pressure. It's not a very pleasant condition, but it's less life-threatening than osteoporosis, in which bones fracture under pressure.

RISK OF OVERDOSE

During growth, as with vitamin A, vitamin D is part of the mechanism to break bone down so that it can then stretch and grow. Thus, an overdose of vitamin D can have the same consequence as vitamin A: breakdown of bone, eventually leading to osteoporosis if unchecked. Overdose cannot occur from exposure to the sun. When the body has manufactured enough D, the mechanism of manufacture is shut down.

VEGAN POINT OF INFORMATION

By law, any milk sold in the United States that is transported across state borders must be fortified with the child's RDA of vitamin D per quart. Thus, an adult, needing less than a child and drinking a quart a day, is getting twice his or her RDA. If that adult also gets any reasonable amount of sun exposure, this double dose represents a triple dose. The very milk that we are being told to drink for strong bones may be contributing toward osteoporosis, the weak-bone disease.

In the 1930s, many cases of rickets were discovered in American school children. Since milk was widely available and being promoted as "healthy" for children, it was decided to use it as the vector for getting extra vitamin D into the children's food supply. Additionally, it was thought that since milk had an abundant supply of calcium, the vitamin D added would help absorb that calcium.

Since that time, it has been discovered that the vitamin D needed to absorb calcium out of the intestine must already be in the bloodstream, meaning the vitamin D in the milk cannot help. Nevertheless, the dairy industry continues to push it as a growth food and now promotes it as an adult food as well. The dairy industry would like everyone to think osteoporosis is caused by deficiencies of calcium and vitamin D (actually, they hope we believe it is caused by a deficiency of cow's milk). It is, however, a condition of excess calcium loss, not deficient intake. As you should now be aware, this loss is contributed to by excess intakes of such substances as protein and vitamins A and D.

VITAMIN E

Also known as **tocopherol**, the most common form being alpha-tocopherol, this vitamin is mainly known for its antioxidant abilities. Recall that unsaturated fatty acids are prone to rancidity by oxidation. It is no coincidence that nature provides ample vitamin E in all foods that contain unsaturated fats. This protects the fats from spoilage in the whole unprocessed food. Trouble only comes when the food is processed in such a way that air can reach the fatty acids. Vitamin E then sacrifices itself to save them. Soon the E is depleted, and then the fat starts to spoil. Since these broken-down products of rancid fats are carcinogenic, vitamin E is considered cancer preventive.

Since there are unsaturated fats in the cell membranes of virtually every type of cell in the body, a severe deficiency of vitamin E can affect every organ system. This is especially true for cells that must replace themselves frequently. In small, highly reproductive animals like rats, sexual cells fall into this category, and so an early sign of vitamin E deficiency in rats is loss of sexual function. Thus, vitamin E gained the notoriety of being an aid to potency and fertility. However, in human beings, much more debilitating effects occur before vitamin E deficiency would affect sexual function, so anyone in otherwise good health who takes vitamin E to improve sexual performance is probably wasting his money.

In human beings it seems that red blood cells (**erythrocytes**) are the first to feel the effects of an E deficiency. (Red blood cells have a short life span and so must be rebuilt frequently.) This loss of integrity of the membranes of these cells is called **erythrocyte hemolysis**.

VITAMIN K

Also known as **phylloquinone** or naphthoquinone, vitamin K is primarily known for its role as one of the factors necessary for blood coagulation after an injury. The letter K was actually given to this vitamin because a Danish researcher discovered it, and the Danish word for coagulation begins with the letter "K." [Note: Many different substances are required for coagulation; people with a disease known as hemophilia lack the ability to manufacture one of the other necessary substances, unrelated to vitamin K.] Vitamin K can be manufactured by bacteria that commonly live in the human intestine. Thus, in most cases, it should not even be considered a vitamin. However, babies are born with a sterile digestive tract and so are frequently given a K injection to prevent excessive bleeding in case of accidental injury. It was formerly thought that human breast milk was a poor source of the vitamin, until it was discovered that a water-soluble form of the vitamin existed in it. It was just not where it was expected to be.

People who are on antibiotic therapy to fight infections often destroy, at least temporarily, the bacteria that manufacture K. For these folks, K becomes a "vitamin" again and must be consumed somehow. Green leafy vegetables are good sources.

Practice Test: UNIT 8 — Fat-Soluble Vitamins

Study the **Information Summary** *and then try to complete this test from memory.**

1. What are the four fat-soluble vitamins?

2. Why are fruits and vegetables safer sources of vitamin A than animal products or supplements?

3. Why do overdoses of vitamins A and D have similar consequences?

4. Which vitamin has been found to help protect lung tissue from the effects of air pollution?

5. Which vitamin is known primarily for its role in blood coagulation after an injury?

6–9.   Match the vitamin with the alternate name of its most common chemical form.

   6. A _____   a. tocopherol

   7. D _____   b. retinol

   8. E _____   c. phylloquinone

   9. K _____   d. calciferol

10. Who needs more vitamin D, children or adults? Why?

*Answer Keys *begin on page 134.*

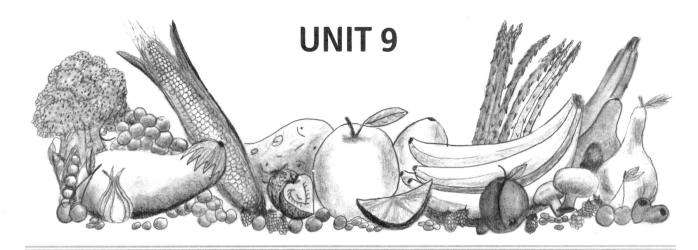

UNIT 9

Water-Soluble Vitamins

Information Summary

The water-soluble vitamins consist of the eight B vitamins and vitamin C.

THE B GROUP

There are eight substances now recognized as B vitamins in the United States. Originally, they were designated by number (B-1, B-2, etc.) but now are usually correctly referred to by their chemical names. (Note that there is a B-12 even though only eight are recognized. This is because some chemicals that function as B vitamins for other animals were found not to apply to human beings and so lost their status, but their numbers were never reassigned, to prevent confusion.) The eight B vitamins are:

1. Thiamin (B-1)   5. Cobalamin (B-12)
2. Riboflavin (B-2)   6. Folacin
3. Niacin (B-3)   7. Pantothenic Acid*
4. Pyridoxine (B-6)   8. Biotin*

[*Deficiencies of these in human beings are virtually impossible because they occur adequately in nearly all foods.]

What these eight have in common is that all contain nitrogen and all function as **coenzymes**. Coenzymes are substances that help enzymes do their work. (The enzymes previously discussed, digestive enzymes, help break things down; there are other enzymes that help build things.)

The difference between enzymes and coenzymes is that the former retain their integrity after doing their work and can be used over and over again. Coenzymes, however, are broken down in the process of doing their work and so must be replaced constantly. Hence, there is a daily need for the water-soluble vitamins, except cobalamin (B-12).

THIAMIN

Beriberi was a crippling disease in southeast Asia in the 1890s. Workers who ate a diet of mostly refined rice lost their ability to perform physical tasks and responded with the words "Beri, beri:" literally, "I can't, I can't." The polishing of rice removed most of its B vitamins, and since the role of one of these (**thiamin** or B-1) is to help burn the calories in carbohydrates, energy levels were drained. This is probably how the myth started that vitamins provide energy. In fact, vitamins provide no calories, but they do permit calories to be liberated from the nutrients that do.

Once whole-grain rice was added back to the diet of these workers, their beriberi subsided. It was theorized at first that the disease was an infectious one and that something in the whole rice (called substance "B" for beriberi) was a curative agent. Years later, thiamin was isolated and was called vital amine B, or vitamin B for short.

RIBOFLAVIN

Sometime after the isolation of thiamin, it was realized that adding this alone back to polished rice did not provide adequate nutrition, and soon **riboflavin** (B-2) was discovered. A lack of this created a condition labeled **ariboflavinosis**, which, among other things, caused cracking at the corners of the mouth. Riboflavin is destroyed by exposure to light. This is why milk was often packaged in brown glass bottles (before the days of plastic), so that when the milkman delivered it and set it on the back porch, the sunlight wouldn't do as much damage.

NIACIN

The third B vitamin discovered was **niacin**. Niacin deficiency is a bit harder to induce because the body can make a certain amount of it from the amino acid tryptophan. **Pellagra** (the niacin deficiency disease) did appear among poor families in the southern United States whose diet was centered on cornmeal and pork fat. Since corn protein is low in tryptophan and pork fat has no protein, niacin could not be manufactured in adequate amounts.

PYRIDOXINE (VITAMIN B-6)

Pyridoxine is deeply involved in amino acid metabolism, so, as you might expect, more is needed as protein intake increases (0.01 mg B-6 per gram of protein is needed). Nature in her wisdom puts abundant B-6 in protein-rich foods (soybeans, nuts, whole grains), although beef and dairy are relatively poor sources.

FOLACIN

Folacin is an important part of red blood cell development, so, as you might expect, a deficiency of it leads to **anemia**. Anemia is an inability of the red blood cells to deliver oxygen to the body, resulting in both physical and mental fatigue. Red blood cells are large when they are first formed and then mature into a smaller, functional size, after which they are filled with hemoglobin, the oxygen-carrying protein. There are two basic types of anemia: one called **macrocytic** ("big cells") and the other called **microcytic** ("small cells"). In microcytic anemia, which is most often caused by a deficiency of the mineral iron and sometimes by lack of pyridoxine (B-6), the red blood cells are smaller than normal because the body cannot manufacture enough hemoglobin. In macrocytic anemia, the red blood cells fail to mature properly, and they remain large and dysfunctional.

COBALAMIN (VITAMIN B-12)

Cobalamin, still most frequently referred to as B-12, has at least two important functions. One is to maintain the integrity of the coating of nerve cells (myelin sheath). The other function is as an activator of folacin in helping mature red blood cells. In regard to the latter function, as you would expect, a cobalamin deficiency leads to the same macrocytic anemia caused by folacin deficiency. The long-term effect of a cobalamin deficiency, though, is degeneration of nerve cells, ultimately leading to paralysis (nerve cells are much longer-living than red blood cells, so problems take longer to develop). Thus, anemia caused by cobalamin deficiency serves as an early warning of nerve damage coming later. Anemia, the caution flag, can be masked, however, by consuming huge doses of folacin. By flooding the body with folacin, enough of it will do its work well enough to overcome the anemia. Thus, the ultimate nerve degeneration will come without further warning; it will start with loss of feeling in the tips of the fingers and toes. Eventually the spine becomes paralyzed, and death results. Anemia caused by lack of cobalamin in the body is referred to as **pernicious anemia** (pernicious meaning "quiet, but deadly"). This is why, by law, folacin-containing supplements cannot contain more than the RDA of folacin in each pill. There is nothing harmful about the excess folacin; it is merely to prevent masking the cobalamin deficiency.

VEGAN POINT OF INFORMATION

There is sometimes worry that the high content of folacin in leafy green vegetables might mask any cobalamin deficiency that vegans may develop. From Table 9.1, it seems it would be easy to far exceed the folacin USRDA of 400 micrograms:

Table 9.1 — Folacin Content of Some Green Vegetables

Vegetable	Folacin (micrograms) per 100 kcal
Spinach, raw	908
Romaine lettuce	844
Spinach, cooked	639
Turnip greens, cooked	590
Iceberg lettuce	430
Broccoli, raw	255
Cabbage, raw	250
Broccoli, cooked	233
Cabbage, cooked	97

One should realize, though, that all of these have very low calorie densities, having much less than one kcal/g. Thus, to consume 100 kcal it is necessary to eat more than 100 grams—usually 300 to 600 grams (remember there are only 454 grams in a pound!). A whole head of iceberg lettuce, for instance, is only about 70 kcal. Cooking does reduce caloric density somewhat (by reducing water content), but it also lowers the vitamin content (much less so in a dense vegetable like broccoli than in leafy ones). In any event, it is important to remember that a high intake of folacin is not harmful in and of itself. In fact, some researchers have correlated low folacin intakes with many common birth defects and recommend huge doses to help prevent them. The wisest course would seem to be a generous but not excessive intake, the latter of which could only be achieved by eating enormous salads at every meal or copious amounts of green vegetable juices.

Other than the B-12 added to certain foods, there are potential sources of cobalamin in the environment. The soil (as well as rain water, sea water, and the atmosphere) is full of the dozens of microorganisms that manufacture cobalamin. Unless one is scrubbing every speck of dirt off vegetables and keeping them tightly sealed until mealtime, there is probably plenty of cobalamin on their surface. In a study published in the journal *Plant and Soil* in 1994, it was shown that although only insignificant quantities of cobalamin are found in plant foods (this study examined soybeans, barley, and spinach) grown in a typical chemically fertilized fashion, the levels of the vitamin increased when organic fertilizer was used.[10]

Furthermore, especially in the case of spinach, the levels increased greatly (to highly nutritionally significant amounts) when pure B-12 was added to the soil. Thus, plants do have the ability to take up this vitamin if the soil is treated properly. It is noteworthy that in some older tables of food composition (prior to 1950), some cobalamin (B-12) is listed as present in fruits such as dates, presumably either because they weren't being scrubbed cleanly enough or more likely because the soils were more organic then. The reality of how people procure and prepare their food before eating it should be considered. Although drops in cobalamin levels do occur when individuals are fed a scrubbed-clean vegan diet, free-living vegans rarely develop a frank deficiency. So who does get a cobalamin deficiency?

First, it must be understood that to absorb cobalamin into the blood from the intestine, a certain carrier molecule must be present in the blood. This carrier, called intrinsic factor (IF), is normally manufactured in the body, but for some unknown reason, certain individuals lose the ability to produce it. It seems to occur most frequently in midlife (age 40 to 50) and mostly among Caucasians. This is by far the most common cause of pernicious anemia, and it occurs in meat eaters and vegans alike (although much more often in meat eaters because there are more of them).

The few cases of diet-induced cobalamin deficiency reported can generally be explained by some anomaly in the individual situation. Some elderly women in England, called "tea and toast ladies," were found to be deficient, probably because their diet provided little opportunity for microorganisms to thrive (they don't do well on hot foods). Some macrobiotic children were found deficient, and this may have been due to the large amounts of sea vegetables consumed by them. It seems that sea vegetables contain some chemicals that are very similar in structure to cobalamin—analogues of it—that are absorbed into the body but fail to do the work. True cobalamin can thus be crowded out, creating a deficiency. In one other case, a 10-month-old infant was being exclusively breast-fed by a vegan mother, and the child exhibited a cobalamin deficiency. At 10 months, the infant should already have been consuming some foods, which would have given him the opportunity for cobalamin ingestion. While breast milk does contain some cobalamin, it is sterile; thus, breast milk is limited in the amount of cobalamin it can provide. It has been shown that the "good" bacteria that thrive in our digestive systems can manufacture cobalamin, although most of it occurs lower in the colon than the normal absorptive sites. Nevertheless, this infant was being denied the ability to grow any such beneficial organisms because his diet was completely sterile.

VITAMIN C

Vitamin C, or ascorbic acid, has received more publicity than any other nutrient, largely due to the research of Linus Pauling on the common cold. Many people probably believe the "C" is meant to stand for "cold." It more appropriately stands for "collagen," the connective tissue of the body that cements everything together. The gums in your mouth are almost pure collagen, and it is no coincidence that bleeding gums are a first sign of C deficiency (although many other conditions can cause bleeding gums).

Vitamin C has many other roles in the body, one of which is its function as an antioxidant (recall that vitamins A and E are the other antioxidant vitamins). These three (actually, vitamin A only in its beta-carotene form) are known as anticancer vitamins, because they will prevent formation of free radicals that result from the oxidative breakdown of fats. How much vitamin C do we need? The answer to that is a good exercise in nutrition recommendation:

- Only about 10 mg/day are needed to prevent scurvy. To be on the safe side, RDAs were originally set at approximately 30 mg, and in the late 1980s, they were raised to a range of 55 to 60 mg to ensure that everyone gets "enough" (overdosing at this level with C is much safer than recommending similar overdoses of, for instance, protein).

- It has been found that tissue saturation occurs at approximately 100 mg/day, meaning that the body just can't hold any more, although smokers reach tissue saturation at as much as 150 mg.

- Symptoms of overdose (diarrhea) don't occur until one reaches a level of approximately 3,000 mg/day.

- Dr. Pauling's recommendations, especially to prevent cancer, are in the range of 10,000 to 12,000 mg a day. He says that patients with cancer do not get diarrhea even at these levels.

- There are reports of pregnant women who habitually take greater than 2,000 mg/day giving birth to infants who develop scurvy unless they (the infants) are given similarly high doses and slowly weaned off them. Obviously, the body becomes habituated to high levels and just doesn't absorb at a normal rate.

DESTRUCTION OF VITAMINS DURING FOOD PREPARATION

Some vitamins are broken down by exposure to stimuli such as air, heat, acids, alkalis, or light. Since most whole foods contain most of the vitamins, it is necessary to try to avoid as many of these factors as possible. Foods should not be cut up until the time of consumption, if possible, and should otherwise be stored in cool, dark places (refrigerators are good). When cooked, exposure to heat should be minimized, although it is difficult to trade off between high temperature and longer cooking time. Microwave ovens seem to destroy no more nutrients than conventional cooking, since cooking time is reduced considerably. Many people avoid microwave ovens, however, because their risk of radiation leakage poses a health hazard if the microwaves are at all damaged.

NOTES

[10] A. Mozafar, "Enrichment of some B-vitamins in plants with application of organic fertilizers," *Plant and Soil* 167, no. 2 (December 1994): 305-311.

Practice Test: UNIT 9 — Water-Soluble Vitamins

Study the **Information Summary** *and then try to complete this test from memory.**

1. Which of the water-soluble vitamins is *not* required from the diet on a daily basis?

2–6. Match the vitamin with its deficiency condition:

_____ 2. Thiamin   a. Scurvy

_____ 3. Riboflavin   b. Pellagra

_____ 4. Niacin   c. Macrocytic anemia

_____ 5. Cobalamin or Folacin   d. Ariboflavinosis

_____ 6. Ascorbic acid   e. Beriberi

7. Describe why the amount of folacin in a supplement is limited by law.

8. Discuss some of the issues relevant to the question "How much vitamin C do I need?"

9. How do you respond to someone who states that a purely vegan diet is inappropriate for human beings because it might lack vitamin B-12?

10. Check the ingredient list on a loaf of "enriched" bread. Which water-soluble vitamins can you recognize?

11. Why do many people believe that vitamins "give you" energy? (Hint: think about beriberi.)

*Answer Keys begin on page 134.

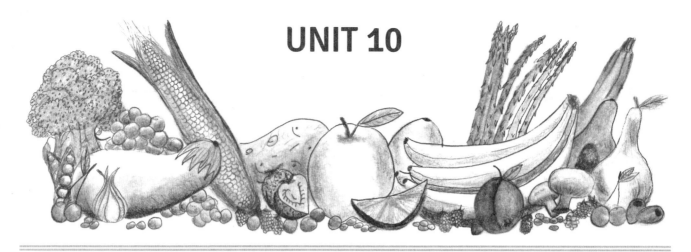

Major Minerals I

Information Summary

OVERVIEW OF MINERALS

Geologically speaking, minerals are the components of rocks. Nutritionally speaking, they are the elements other than carbon, hydrogen, oxygen, and nitrogen that we need to obtain from our diets. Any other elements that may appear in food are considered **inert material** and sometimes are referred to as **contaminants** if they are toxic at relatively low levels. To demonstrate how new and inexact a science nutrition is, consider that not too long ago copper was considered a contaminant. We now know that it is needed in tiny amounts, so it is now considered a "mineral."

Minerals are categorized into two groups, based on the amounts we need in the diet:

> **Major Minerals**: Adult need of 100 mg or more per day
> **Trace Minerals**: Adult need of 50 mg or less per day

There are seven major minerals: calcium, phosphorus, magnesium, sulfur, sodium, potassium, and chlorine. The first four will be discussed in this chapter; the latter three and water will be discussed in Unit 11. The 10 or so (the inexactness of this number is a further reflection of the newness of nutrition as a science) trace minerals are discussed in Unit 12.

Remember that minerals are all inorganic nutrients. They do not provide calories, nor can they be broken down or created in any animal or plant body. They must ultimately come from the earth, from which they are taken up into plants, and those plants are then eaten by animals. In food preparation, minerals cannot be destroyed, but they can be removed (by milling off outer layers, for instance) or can leach out into the water that foods are soaked or cooked in. If soaked out, the water they are soaked in will always contain what is missing, so they can still be consumed as a broth.

Since minerals are part of rocks and are plentiful in soil, the body has a way of preventing overdose from accidental ingestion (a common occurrence among dirt- and sand-eating kids). The absorption from the digestive tract into the bloodstream is limited. Usually certain carrier molecules must be available or the minerals are left to pass through the tract and out in the feces. For some minerals, such as calcium and iron, absorption can be as low as 1% and is rarely as high as 30%. Absorption of other minerals, such as sodium and potassium (which can be excreted more easily through urine), is usually in the 70%–95% range.

MINERALS & FIBER

You are already aware that excess fiber can inhibit mineral absorption by pushing the food material too quickly through the digestive tract, thereby shortening the exposure of the minerals to the intestinal wall. There is another issue that gives fiber bad press in relation to mineral absorption, and that is the presence of chemical binders in the fiber of certain foods. These binders have the potential to attach themselves to minerals (especially calcium, iron, and zinc) and render them unable to be absorbed by the body, such that they are passed out in the feces. The most notorious of these binders are phytic acid (found in most whole grains) and oxalic acid (particularly present in spinach and rhubarb). While the effects of these are potentially significant, they seem to show up more often under laboratory conditions than they do in the real world. It is likely that foods also contain enzymes that break down these binders and force them to release at least part of the minerals for absorption. It is known, for example, that when whole grain flour is combined with yeast in the making of bread, the yeast inactivates the phytic acid. The only population of people that seemed to have a problem with binders was in the Middle East (Egypt) where whole wheat crackers without yeast are a staple of the diet.

THE MAJOR MINERALS

There are seven major minerals: **calcium**, **phosphorus**, **magnesium**, **sulfur**, **sodium**, **potassium**, and **chlorine**.

CALCIUM (Ca)

A large part of the calcium story is already known to you: its loss from the body from excess protein, vitamin A, or vitamin D intake and the body's inability to absorb calcium when vitamin D is deficient.

The typical adult body contains approximately 1,200 grams (almost 3 lbs) of calcium, 99% of it being in the bones and teeth. It is the other 1% in the blood that tries to maintain itself in a fairly constant state and steals from the great storage in the bones when needed. The calcium in the blood is necessary for nerve impulse transmission and muscle contraction. A shortage naturally causes serious damage, such as the cessation of heartbeat.

The recommended intake of calcium in the United States is much higher than it is for less affluent populations. This is because it is assumed that Americans consume a large amount of protein and thus need more calcium to help make up for its incurred loss. Not only is this an absurd approach to plug up a problem, it does not work very well either. Usually only 10%–30% of the calcium in foods commonly eaten in the United States (this applies to beverages such as milk as well) is absorbed into the bloodstream from the intestine by adults. The remaining calcium in the foods is excreted in the feces. However, growing children generally absorb 50%–60%, as do pregnant women. Obviously, the body has the wisdom to know when it needs more of this bone-growing material. The fact that people with osteoporosis do not absorb calcium at the higher level is indicative of the fact that there is no *deficiency* perceived. In the June 1997 issue of the *American Journal of Public Health*, researchers from Harvard School of Public Health published "Milk, Dietary Calcium, and Bone Fractures in Women: A 12-Year Prospective Study."[11] This article concludes that women who drink two or more glasses of milk a day have no fewer (actually slightly higher) risk of hip fractures than those who drink one glass or less. This is in spite of the fact that the extra calcium may increase *overall bone mass*. This measurement apparently does not equate with increased *bone strength*.

A true deficiency of calcium results in the same disorders as vitamin D deficiency: **rickets** in children and **osteomalacia** in adults. Since vitamin D is necessary for absorption of calcium from the intestine, a lack of either one logically will have the same consequences. The *loss* of calcium from bone, observed in osteoporosis, is a different phenomenon.

Indiscriminate supplementation with calcium pills has its risks: an *excess intake* of calcium can lead to kidney stone formation, at least in some people who are genetically predisposed to it. Also, since many minerals are absorbed at the same sites in the intestine, flooding the digestive system with some of them can inhibit absorption of others. It has been found that taking large amounts of certain calcium supplements interferes with magnesium absorption. Yet when magnesium is also added to the calcium supplement, iron absorption is inhibited. Best to let nature alone and just not consume the excess protein that prompts the additional calcium in the first place.

CALCIUM SOURCES

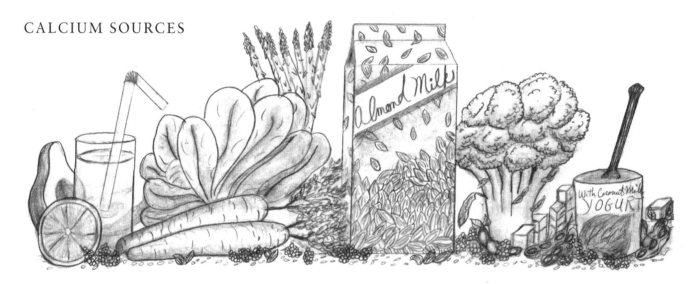

VEGAN POINT OF INFORMATION

While food sources of nutrients will be discussed in the subsequent chapters on vegan foods, it is worth dwelling on non-animal sources of calcium to allay fears that a pure vegan diet may be lacking in this mineral. All one need do is ponder where cows get their calcium from to put into their milk to realize that green plants are abundant in this very common element. Again, no animal can manufacture any mineral; it must come from its diet. (And no adult cows drink milk or take calcium supplements.) One cup of broccoli, for instance, has nearly 200 mg of calcium, which is approximately the adult minimum daily need. The FAO/WHO recommendations are 350 mg daily just to be generously on the safe side. The USRDA has traditionally been 800 mg to help make up for our high protein diet, and now it may be raised to 1,200 mg because Americans have been eating more protein than ever.

THE "VITAMIN D & CALCIUM IN MILK" ISSUE

The fact that milk was chosen as the vector to deliver vitamin D to any potentially sun-starved children does *not* make it a better source of calcium (dairy commercials may still try to claim otherwise). It has since been discovered that the vitamin D necessary to absorb the calcium moving down the intestine must already have been in the bloodstream for a while; what is present with that calcium is useless at that stage.

PHOSPHORUS (P)

Phosphorus has several roles to play in the body. One is as an antagonist to calcium in the blood. The concentration of calcium multiplied by the concentration of phosphorus tends to remain as a constant number. Thus, as the calcium level in the blood rises, the phosphorous level falls, and vice versa. So an excess intake of phosphorus can be added to the list of things that cause a loss of calcium from the blood and eventually from the bones. Meats are particularly rich in phosphorus and very deficient in calcium. Many soft drinks (like Coke, Pepsi, etc.) have **phosphoric acid** as an ingredient and are totally devoid of calcium. The great American lunch, a hamburger and a Coke, is no friend to your skeleton.

MAGNESIUM (Mg)

Magnesium is the central atom in the chlorophyll molecule. (Chlorophyll has a structure remarkably similar to hemoglobin in blood, with one significant difference being that an iron atom occupies the central position in the latter). In human beings, magnesium plays several important roles: it contributes to strong tooth and bone structure, helps release calories from energy-containing molecules, and is necessary for nerve impulse transmission.

Deficiencies of magnesium have been known to occur in people suffering severe vomiting and/or chronic diarrhea, as well as in alcohol abusers. There is no name for the deficiency, but it usually causes weakness, confusion, and sometimes convulsions and hallucinations. In children, growth failure can result. Toxic effects from excess intake only seem to cause diarrhea. The medicine Epsom salts (a magnesium salt), usually employed as a soaking agent, is sometimes used as a laxative.

SULFUR (S)

Sulfur meets the definition of a major mineral, yet attention is generally not paid to it. Since sulfur is contained in the essential amino acid **methionine** (as well as in two nonessential amino acids), it is impossible to incur a sulfur deficiency without also having a protein deficiency. Sulfur is also present in the B vitamins thiamin and biotin.

VEGAN POINT OF INFORMATION

Animal products are rich in the sulfur-containing amino acids, the smell of rotting eggs being a testament to this. It has been demonstrated that when these amino acids are deaminated, the waste products have more affinity for carrying out calcium than any of the other amino acids. Thus, animal protein does more damage to bone structure than an equal amount of plant protein.

NOTES

[11] D. Feskanich et al., "Milk, Dietary Calcium, and Bone Fractures in Women: A 12-Year Prospective Study," *American Journal of Public Health* 87, no. 6 (June 1997): 992-997.

Practice Test: UNIT 10 — Major Minerals I

Study the **Information Summary** *and then try to complete this test from memory.**

1. What are the differences between vitamins and minerals?

2. How are major minerals distinguished from trace minerals?

3. Why is the recommended calcium intake so much higher in the USA than in less affluent countries?

4. The normal adult absorbs about what percent of the calcium present in foods eaten?

    a. 10%–30%   b. 60%–80%   c. 90%   d. 100%

5. Describe the difference between osteoporosis and osteomalacia, especially as related to dietary indiscretions.

6. What are chemical binders in foods, and what is their nutritional significance?

7. What do you say to someone who insists human beings need milk for strong bones because it is the only reliable source of calcium and vitamin D?

8. How does meat consumption contribute to poor calcium status? (List at least two ways.)

9. What is the central atom in chlorophyll molecules?

10. Why is a deficiency of sulfur in and of itself not a likely occurrence?

*Answer Keys *begin on page 134.*

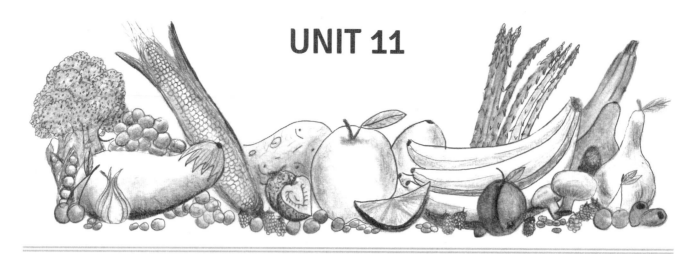

UNIT 11

Major Minerals II & Water

Information Summary

The other three major minerals have much to do with fluid balance in the body, so a brief discussion of water, the most overlooked nutrient, will be included in this chapter.

SALTS & ELECTROLYTES

The word "salt" is colloquially used to refer to sodium chloride, the two-atom molecules that compose common table salt, whether mined from rocks or evaporated from sea water (actually, all rock salt is a result of sea water dried up long ago). The chemist's definition of a salt, however, is any compound other than acids and bases that is composed of ions (charged atoms or molecules). Since these charged particles, such as sodium ($Na+$) and chloride ($Cl-$), dissociate in water (at which point they are called electrolytes) and since water molecules tend to cluster around these ions, they tend to act as "magnets" for water. Thus, if you put some fresh lettuce in a salty dressing, in an hour or so the lettuce will have wilted because its purer water was pulled out into the saltier environment. For nutrition purposes, then, the significance of any salt is its tendency to attract water *to* wherever the salt is present in a higher concentration *from* a solution in which it is in a lower concentration. This flow of water in the body is accomplished because the membranes surrounding each cell are selectively permeable; that is, they allow water to move freely but do not admit dissolved materials.

Positively-charged particles are called cations; negative ones are called anions (not to be confused with onions, although the latter may have a negative effect on your social life). The body maintains electric neutrality, so there is always a balance between these two. The fluid inside body cells is called **intracellular** fluid; the fluid outside is **extracellular** (or **interstitial**) fluid. There are several different ions present in each of these fluid mixtures, but the principal ones are:

> Intracellular: Cation – Potassium   Anion – Phosphate
> Extracellular: Cation – Sodium   Anion – Chloride

Each cell, then, is surrounded by a salt water solution (sodium chloride) that is supposedly similar in concentration to the ancient oceans that once covered the earth. Evolutionists believe this was the way land animals adapted for survival. (Present-day oceans are actually quite a bit saltier than this, though, so don't try drinking sea water to quench your thirst—it won't work.)

SODIUM (Na)

Many people believe sodium is an unnecessary, unhealthful component of food, similar to cholesterol or saturated fat in that regard. On the contrary, sodium is indeed an essential nutrient and must be included in the diet on a regular basis. Sodium is the principal cation in extracellular fluid and thus helps maintain fluid balance and provides part of the electrical current necessary for impulse transmission. It is also a component of sodium bicarbonate, the pancreatic secretion that neutralizes the stomach acid as the chyme enters the duodenum and creates an alkaline medium in which most digestive enzymes do their best work. It is, however, abundant in foods, beverages, and even water (especially so-called "softened" water).

Table salt is 40% sodium by weight. Thus, one gram of salt contains 400 mg of sodium. A teaspoon of salt weighs approximately 5 g and contains approximately 2,000 mg of sodium (5 g = 5,000 mg; 40% of 5,000 = 2,000). The minimum requirement of human adults for sodium is, at most, approximately 115 mg/day. This is the amount that is present in approximately 300 mg of salt (40% of 300 = about 115), approximately one-fifteenth of a teaspoon. The Canadian government recommends this amount as a minimum requirement. Legislators in the United States are much more prone to pressures from food industries such as lobbyists from the snack food associations and the dairy industry. Most dairy products, especially cheeses, are loaded with salt. The "minimum" is set at a generous 500 mg sodium, an amount present in 1,250 mg of salt (about one-fourth teaspoon). Since most Americans now consume approximately four times this amount, the official "recommendation" (although technically not an RDA) of the National Research Council is to "limit daily salt intake to less than 6 grams." This amount contains a whopping 2,400 mg of Na, more than 20 times the minimum requirement, and is one of the more blatant examples of bowing to food industry pressure to maintain the status quo.

It has been reported that excess sodium pulls out calcium into the urine.[12] Thus, similar to the effects of moderating protein, reducing sodium to moderate levels can prevent the bone loss of osteoporosis.

CHLORIDE (Cl)

The other 60% of table salt is chloride (Cl–). Like sodium, chloride is often overlooked as an essential nutrient because more than enough is present in any typical diet. Just a few years ago, however, some baby formula had to be taken off the market because the chloride content was left too low, causing serious illness.

Chloride is the ionic form of the element **chlorine** (Cl_2), which is a poisonous gas. (The latter is what is commonly added to public water supplies, although it is supposed to be fully evaporated before we drink it.) The chloride form is not poisonous, of course, yet in excess may contribute to high blood pressure.

As the chief extracellular anion, chloride helps maintain fluid balance. It is also a component of hydrochloric acid, secreted by the stomach to help break apart proteins. Chloride requirements are set to correspond with those of sodium because they usually occur together. In Canada, the minimum requirement is set at 175 mg/day for adults (the amount found in 300 mg of salt). In the United States, the "minimum" requirement is estimated at 750 mg (amount present in one-fourth teaspoon of salt).

Usually the body loses sodium and chloride together (that is why sweat is salty). An exception to this is during severe vomiting, when the contents of the stomach, containing significant amounts of hydrochloric acid, are lost. Sodium bicarbonate, the digestive juice that contains sodium, enters the digestive tract lower down in the small intestine and so is not lost through vomitus.

POTASSIUM (K)

Potassium is the chief cation inside the cells. Like the other electrolytes, it plays an important role in transmission of nerve and muscle contractions. An overload of potassium will stop the heart by not allowing it to relax.

When people retain water abnormally (a condition called edema), high blood pressure is sometimes the result. When diuretics (substances that cause the body to excrete water) are given, many of them work by fooling the body into thinking there is a deficiency of sodium. The kidneys react by withholding sodium and excreting water in order to raise the relative concentration of sodium. This excreted water always has a certain concentration of ions in it, but the kidneys make sure that the cations to be lost are K+, not Na+. So along with the water, potassium is lost. To replenish it, foods need to be eaten that have lots of potassium but not too much sodium (the body is already retaining more than it normally would want to). To begin with, the minimum requirement for potassium is approximately 2,000 mg daily, at least four times greater than that of sodium. So a key number to look at in food composition is the potassium-to-sodium ratio, seeking to achieve a value of 4:1 or higher.

VEGAN POINT OF INFORMATION

Most vegetables have a K:Na ratio greater than 10:1. High-sodium vegetables such as celery and Swiss chard are still up around 3:1. The ratio of most fruits (and even many vegetables, especially those that are botanically fruits, such as eggplant and squash) is greater than 100:1, with grains at approximately 50:1. Animal products are a nightmare: a typical hamburger has a ratio of 0.5:1; bacon is 0.2:1; and American cheese is 0.1:1! Most people believe that bananas are the best source of potassium; many actually think they are the only source. Not so. On a calorie-for-calorie basis, mushrooms are probably the best source, and tomatoes, potatoes, green beans, and strawberries all exceed the level found in bananas.

HUMANITARIAN POINT OF INFORMATION

The reason this banana issue is mentioned is a sociopolitical one. Most of the bananas eaten in the United States, Canada, and Europe come from hungry countries in the tropics that use their best farmland for growing cash crops like bananas (and sugar, coffee, tea, and even flowers) instead of food for local consumption. The result is malnutrition and political unrest, along with the sorrow of attempted illegal emigration to follow their food. It seems appropriate that vegans who wish to make the world a kinder, gentler place would not contribute to this human injustice. The other, better sources of potassium mentioned above all grow quite well in the temperate climates in which we live, and our struggling farmers will also appreciate our helping keep them in business. It is a sad testament indeed to the worsening nature of this problem that just a few years ago bananas replaced good old "American-as-mom" apples as the #1 consumed fruit in the United States.

WATER (H_2O)

Adult human beings are typically 55%–60% water by weight. On an average day, approximately two and a half quarts are excreted through the kidneys (urine), skin (perspiration), lungs (water vapor in expired breath), and digestive tract (feces) combined. This same amount is taken in through food and drink, although a small amount (approximately a half cup) is created as a byproduct of metabolism (burning calories). Even in the absence of any water intake, approximately a pint must be excreted each day (obligatory water loss) to rid the body of wastes. Death from dehydration would follow in just a few days if this were not replaced. Even at a mere pint, water is still the essential nutrient needed in largest quantity.

Approximately eight quarts of water are cycled through the digestive tract each day, turning digesting food into liquid chyme. Normally all except one-fourth cup of this water is reabsorbed through the colon and put back into circulation. Imagine how quickly one can become dehydrated when diarrhea allows significantly more water to be eliminated. Children are hardest hit by this effect.

Water is often categorized as *soft* or *hard*. Hard water (sometimes called well water) usually has significant amounts of calcium and magnesium in it. These minerals do not allow soap (and consequently dirt) to be dissolved very well. Thus, many people soften their water for washing purposes by adding some form of salt (often containing sodium) to it. For drinking purposes, though, hard water is preferable because it contains minerals that people usually don't get enough of (it usually tastes better, too), whereas soft water contains one mineral of which they usually get too much.

VEGAN POINT OF INFORMATION

Most meats are 55%–60% water (just like us). Although some may say that this justifies it as an appropriate "food," the fact that we normally excrete so much water each day makes it much more appropriate that we eat foods with a higher water content than our bodies have. Just eating meat would leave no extra fluid, thereby obliging us to drink more water. This may be no pure rationale for veganism, but because it is getting harder and harder to find pure, unpolluted water, any diet that obliges us to find more of it is a minus in that regard. It is indeed ironic that the livestock industry is responsible for more water pollution in the United States than all other sources of pollution combined.

NOTES

[12] Lynda A. Frassetto et al., "Adverse Effects of Sodium Chloride on Bone in the Aging Human Population Resulting from Habitual Consumption of Typical American Diets," *Journal of Nutrition* 138, no. 2 (February 2008) 419S–422S.

Practice Test: UNIT 11 — Major Minerals II & Water

Study the **Information Summary** *and then try to complete this test from memory.**

1. Why does lettuce wilt if left in a salty solution?

2. The principal ions inside and outside human cells are:

   Inside + =   Inside - =

   Outside + =   Outside - =

3. Which of the following are essential nutrients? *(circle one)*

   Water   Sodium   Chloride   Cholesterol   Salt

4. By weight, what percent of table salt is sodium? What percent is chloride?

5. Which digestive fluids contain each of these?

   Na:

   Cl:

6. The need for potassium is about how many times the need for sodium?

   a. one half   b. the same as   c. twice   d. four times

7. People on certain diuretic medications are told to increase their potassium intake. Why?

Practice Test: UNIT 11 — Major Minerals II & Water

8. Name three vegan foods richer in potassium than bananas:

9. About what percent of human body weight is water?

    a. 5%   b. 15%   c. 55%   d. 95%

10. How much is the obligatory water loss of human adults each day?

    a. one tablespoon   b. one cup   c. one pint   d. one gallon

11. How much water is cycled through the digestive tract each day?

    a. two cups   b. two pints   c. two quarts   d. two gallons

12. Most fruits and vegetables are about what percent water by weight?

    a. 5%–10%   b. 15%–25%   c. 45%–55%   d. 85%–95%

13. Meat is about what percent water?

    a. 5%–10%   b. 15%–25%   c. 55%–60%   d. 85%–95%

14. Discuss why the water content of fruits and vegetables is more appropriate to human nutrition than that of meats.

15. A typical fast-food fish sandwich has 150 mg potassium and 750 mg sodium. What is its K:Na ratio, and how might you respond, in this regard, to someone who asks, "It's fish...it's good for you, isn't it?"

*Answer Keys *begin on page 134.*

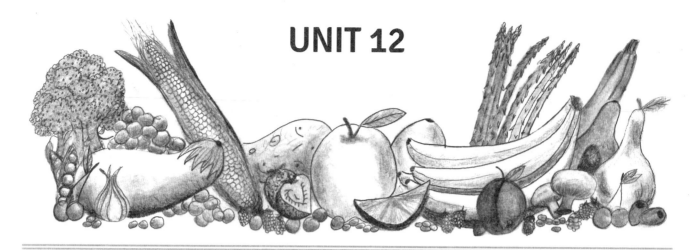

UNIT 12

Trace Minerals

Trace minerals are those that are required in amounts of less than 50 mg/day by human adults. There are nine elements thus regarded: iron, iodine, zinc, copper, manganese, chromium, selenium, molybdenum, and fluoride. A tenth, cobalt (a part of the cobalamin [vitamin B-12] molecule), is listed as a trace mineral in some sources. Since deficiency is said only to occur if B-12 is deficient, cobalt is often not considered as a separate nutrient.

RECOMMENDED DAILY ALLOWANCES (RDA) & ESADDI

The official United States government recommendations for most of the major nutrients are given as Recommended Daily Allowances (RDA), considered to be the average need of healthy individuals consuming a typical diet. For many of the trace minerals, however, there is no scientific consensus as yet on just how much is needed. This is because some trace minerals are only newly recognized as essential nutrients and also because some are needed in such minute amounts that measurement of them is extremely difficult. For these nutrients, the National Research Council has set up Estimated Safe and Adequate Daily Dietary Intakes (ESADDI), broad ranges within which the average need probably falls. These ranges are usually estimated according to what typical intakes are of people who show no signs of deficiency or toxicity of the nutrient in question. Since some of these are very toxic in larger quantities, often more is known about the safe upper limit than about the lower limit, or minimum need, which may be minute.

SOIL DEPLETION & TRACE MINERALS

Many people take supplements of nutrients on the premise that our soils are depleted from decades of overfarming. There may be some truth to this with regard to some trace minerals, but overall, the reasoning is faulty. Consider that in some of the poorer countries of the world, heavy population density makes overfarming mandatory. It is documented in Pakistan, for instance, that the same parcels of land have been used to grow the same crops by the progeny of the same families for more than 3,000 years (!) with no loss of nutrients that anyone can notice. In the United States and Canada, probably no land has been tilled continuously for even one-tenth of that time. Yet we do indeed have some pretty barren soils. The difference is, of course, what is put back on the land after each harvest. People in Pakistan may recycle everything (including their own wastes) back into the soil. We have always dumped everything into landfills or out into waterways. Many of us are finally catching on to the dual advantages of composting our wastes and returning them to the garden: less pollution and better soil. There have been several analyses done on organically grown produce versus chemically grown produce, and usually the former have at least slightly higher contents of most nutrients, particularly the trace minerals. One of the reasons for this is that one of the common fertilizers used on organic produce is seaweed extract. The oceans contain all known trace minerals, and our years of dumping wastes into them have likely added to the pool. Using these fertilizing extracts is probably the safest way to reclaim them. Those who advocate eating fish or other "seafood" obtain not only a huge dose of protein without fiber, but also a heavy contamination of all the toxic materials being dumped into waterways as well. Eating sea plants themselves, a truer sea "food," is certainly better (less protein, lots of fiber, less toxicity, being lower in the food pyramid/chain), but contamination is still possible, and problems like vitamin B-12 analogues may occur. Using these plants as fertilizers allows land plants to selectively filter in the beneficial elements while excluding toxic ones through their root system. Another approach used is to process sewage sludge for composting.

The drawbacks of relying on supplements are discussed below, especially in the section on zinc. Our knowledge of human nutrition, particularly regarding trace minerals, is far from complete.

IRON (Fe)

The most well-known and well-studied of the trace minerals, iron is found in every living cell on earth. It is also one of the most abundant elements in the earth's crust, soil being full of it. It is indeed ironic (excuse the pun) that it is considered the number one problem nutrient in human diets. Estimates are that about 20% of all women and approximately 3% of all men in the United States and Canada are iron deficient. The rates in most poorer countries are judged to be even higher.

Why should women be iron deficient more often than men? The answer lies in a principal role of iron in the body as a central atom in the hemoglobin molecule, which carries oxygen in the blood. Oxygen is necessary for the cells of the body to burn glucose, their preferred energy source. Without enough hemoglobin, which cannot be made without enough iron, every cell in the body fatigues easily, so the classic tiredness of anemia from iron-poor blood results. Because iron is so important, the body holds dearly onto what it has. Daily losses from urine and shed skin cells amount to barely 1 mg in human adults. Whenever blood is lost, however, much iron is lost as well. (About 80% of the total iron in the body is tied up in hemoglobin in the blood). During a woman's monthly menstrual cycle, approximately 15 mg of iron is lost. If this is not made up for in the ensuing month, the depletion continues and thus worsens the iron status. Averaged over a 30-day month, this 15 mg loss only figures out to $15 \div 30 = 0.5$ mg a day. This, in addition to the 1 mg lost to urine and shed skin (which goes on all the time), means that a woman's need for iron averages 1.5 mg daily, compared to an adult male's need of 1.0 mg. Thus, the RDA for women (15 mg) is higher than for men (10 mg). Both these numbers reflect an assumption of 10% absorbability for the iron consumed: 10% of 15 = 1.5 mg absorbed; 10% of 10 = 1.0 mg absorbed. This difference in need between the sexes may not seem like much, but consider that most women are smaller in stature and thus need fewer calories each day. Their foods, then, must be much more nutrient dense with respect to iron to meet their higher requirement.

Compounding this is the fact that dairy foods are notoriously poor in iron, and women are being encouraged to drink more milk to "get their calcium." It is still frequently stated that vegetarians tend to become anemic. The basis for this is that flesh foods are an abundant source of iron and that most vegetarians continue to consume dairy products, often at an increased level. Many vegetarian entrees are loaded with cheese, and many vegetarians feel this is the best way to get their nutrients in the absence of meat. Iron status will suffer greatly, however. Eggs do not offer an acceptable alternative, either, because their moderate iron content is very poorly absorbed.

Iron exists in two forms: the ferric ($Fe+3$) and the ferrous ($Fe+2$) form. The latter is much better absorbed. Certain constituents of foods, especially ascorbic acid, will change ferric iron to ferrous iron, rendering it more absorbable. A third form of iron, just plain elemental iron (Fe), is what cast-iron pots are made of, and it is the least absorbable of all (thankfully, or anyone using cast iron would soon suffer from iron overload). Acid foods do help here, too, as tomato sauce cooked in cast iron has up to 25 times the iron content as that cooked in any other type of pot.

By law, any grain product (flour, rice, cereals, etc.) labeled "enriched" must have iron and the B vitamins thiamin, niacin, and riboflavin added to them in amounts that approximate the original unrefined grain. Some say that because the refined products have had fiber, along with any associated chemical binders (such as phytates), removed the minerals they do have will be better absorbed. Unfortunately, iron is the only mineral added, and most other minerals (and vitamins) are lost in the milling process. The loss of the benefits of fiber makes this an even poorer trade-off.

VEGAN POINT OF INFORMATION

There is often much attention paid to the absorbability of heme vs. non-heme iron. Heme iron (as contained in hemoglobin and the closely related molecule myoglobin) is found in animal flesh. It is absorbed at an average rate of 23%, compared to an average of approximately 10% for non-heme iron, yet heme iron only constitutes 40% of the iron in animal flesh. The other 60% is non-heme iron. Thus, the overall absorption of iron from flesh is 40% × 23% = 9.3% + 60% × 10% = 6% for a total of 15.3%.

Ascorbic acid (or vitamin C, as you all hopefully know by now) enhances non-heme iron absorption, often to levels approaching 20%. To achieve this, more than 100 mg of ascorbic acid must be present in the meal. This is not an inordinate amount if a significant amount of fresh fruits and/or vegetables are included. Thus, the iron in a meal rich in vitamin C may be better absorbed than that in a meat-centered meal.

TOO MUCH IRON?

While intake of too much of any nutrient can be harmful (in the case of iron, this rare condition is called **iron overload**), two studies published in 1994 indicated that high iron intakes may also increase both heart attack and cancer risk, our two most common killer diseases. In the American Heart Association journal *Circulation*, researchers at Harvard University looked at nearly 45,000 men and found that the more heme iron (the kind from flesh foods) consumed, the greater the incidence of heart attack—discounting, of course, the effect of the saturated fat and cholesterol.[13] In that same year, the *International Journal of Cancer* reported a study in which more than 41,000 men and women were studied over 14 years and found to have three times the colon and rectal cancer incidence if their blood iron levels were high.[14]

On the topic of iron overload and cancer, Melodie Anne Coffman, a nutrition consultant, wrote this in 2011:

Heme iron, which is more bioavailable in your body, is found in animal foods, such as beef, poultry and fish. Your body can efficiently absorb 15 percent to 35 percent of the heme iron you consume from your diet, explains the Office of Dietary Supplements. Nonheme iron, from plants, fortified foods and supplements, relies on several factors before it can be absorbed. For example, vitamin C increases the absorption of nonheme iron, while calcium can inhibit absorption. Depending on other foods in your diet, you only absorb 2 percent to 20 percent of nonheme iron you ingest. Since bioavailability of each type of iron is different, they can each have varying effects on cancer risk. Heme iron seems to increase cancer risk due to its ability to be absorbed easily into the bloodstream.... Research published in the "Nutrition and Cancer" journal in 2005 evaluated the effects of heme iron and other nutrients in relation to lung cancer. Although you need iron for oxygen transport, it acts like a pro-oxidant in your body, providing breeding grounds for free radicals to jump in and damage cells. Some iron is stored in the tissues surrounding lungs, leading to possible damage from free radicals. Ingesting foods rich in heme iron can increase your risk of lung cancer, which decreases when combined with a zinc-rich diet. Zinc is an antioxidant that can fight off free radicals that expand with high iron intake. A diet high in heme iron foods such as animal meat may increase your risk of lung cancer, but this type of diet is also high in unhealthy fats which increases your risk of obesity and many types of cancer.[15]

IODINE (I)

The principal role of iodine in the human body is as a part of the thyroid hormones, one of which—thyroxin—regulates the basal metabolic rate. A deficiency of iodine causes an enlargement of the thyroid gland located in the neck, a condition known as goiter. This occurs because the cells of the gland seek to trap as much iodine as they can, and they increase their odds by getting bigger. Two other things can cause goiter. First, chemicals called goitrogens that occur in some plants that are eaten in certain parts of Africa block the effectiveness of thyroxin in the body. The second cause of goiter, oddly enough, is overconsumption of iodine.

Iodine is found in plant foods grown in soil rich in iodine. This excludes certain areas around the Great Lakes and in eastern Oregon. To help these people avoid deficiency, it was decided to fortify salt with iodine many years ago. Since that time, salt consumption, especially that added to fast foods, has risen tremendously. Iodine is also present in some baked goods that have iodate dough conditioners added during processing. The third, and most insidious, source of iodine contamination is through dairy products. Dairy cows are subject to an infection of the udders known as mastitis. The usual treatment for this is a swabbing of iodine antiseptic. Apparently, significant amounts of this iodine are found in the milk supply. At the present time in the United States, risk of overconsumption of iodine is probably greater than risk of deficiency.

ZINC

Zinc (Zn) has so many functions in the human body that it is hard to believe it was largely ignored as a nutrient until the 1960s. That was when the first cases of human zinc deficiency were reported. Among some people in the Middle East (Egypt, Iran, Turkey), a staple of the diet is unleavened (baked without yeast) whole-grain wheat bread. The chemical binders, called phytates, present in these whole grains were thus not broken down during the yeast fermentation process as they are in the breads consumed elsewhere. Zinc absorption was impaired, and the deficiency manifested itself as growth retardation and delayed sexual development in young males. The classic photograph in nutrition textbooks is of a seventeen-year-old boy with the appearance of a seven-year-old. Since subsequent zinc supplementation brought on a resumption of normal growth and development, the conclusion was that these people suffered a true deficiency of this mineral. When this became popularized in the press, the sexual maturation issue was highlighted, and zinc became the "wonder cure" for any male sexual problems. Although it is true that a zinc deficiency can cause delayed sexual development and decreased sperm production, it does not cure impotence or any other sexual problem in men with normal zinc status. Yet millions were spent on zinc supplements anyway.

In the early 1980s, a report was published proclaiming that large doses of zinc could shorten the duration of the common cold. Subsequent studies have failed to confirm this, yet—again—sales of zinc supplements were boosted further. This extra supplementation did result in two conclusions: first, that high-level intake of zinc could lower the HDL-cholesterol level (the "good" kind), thereby possibly raising risk of heart disease. It is interesting to note that a deficiency of zinc also tends to promote atherosclerosis. Like some other nutrients (such as iodine and vitamin D), too little or too much zinc causes similar damaging effects. Secondly, some people taking high doses of zinc developed an anemia not responsive to iron, folacin, or cobalamin. Eventually it was discovered that these people were deficient in copper, an element not previously thought to be essential to human nutrition. It seems that the small amount of copper people do need to absorb was being crowded out by all the zinc present in the digestive tract. Many of the trace minerals are absorbed at the same intestinal sites, so overload of one can greatly decrease the ability of the body to absorb one or more of the others. This demonstrated very clearly the need for balance in the diet and the danger of oversupplementation.

Galvanized metals are coated with a zinc-containing material and can sometimes be a source of excessive intake as well. Since zinc is closely associated with many proteins in nature, foods that are highest in protein are usually highest in zinc content. Because of the potential problem with chemical binders in grains, the usual recommendation is to seek animal protein as an assurance of adequate zinc intake. It should be clear, however, that yeast-leavened grain products are good sources of zinc because the yeast inactivates the phytates (through the production of phytases, enzymes that break them apart). Nuts, vegetables, legumes, and seeds—especially pumpkin seeds—are excellent sources of zinc as well. Usually approximately 20% of the zinc in food is absorbed. The United States RDA for zinc is 12 mg for women and 15 mg for men. In Canada, the recommendations are 9 and 12 mg, respectively.

VEGAN POINT OF INFORMATION

With all the attention paid to the inhibition of zinc absorption by the phytates in grain, another inhibitor of zinc absorption is often ignored: casein, the primary protein in cow's milk. The primary protein in human breast milk is alpha-lactalbumin, which does not have this effect and is more easily digested.

COPPER

As mentioned above, the role of copper in human nutrition only began to be discerned after people overdosing on zinc created a copper-deficient state in their blood. It is now known that copper (Cu) serves as a catalyst in the formation of hemoglobin, and so a deficiency in copper causes a microcytic anemia that does not respond to iron. Only 2 mg of copper are needed daily and can be easily obtained from grains, nuts, and seeds (remarkably similar sources to that of zinc: nature puts them together so they won't out-compete each other). Copper plumbing pipes and copper cookware are possible sources of excess intake, and care should be taken not to frequently consume water that has been standing in these pipes for long periods and to minimize time of food contact with copper utensils. Toxicity can occur at intakes of as little as 10 mg daily. Symptoms usually include vomiting and diarrhea.

MANGANESE

Not to be confused with the major mineral magnesium, manganese (Mn) has only been recognized as an essential nutrient since the 1970s. It is now known that it has several functions, despite the fact that less than 20 mg are normally present in the adult body. An intake of 3 mg per day is considered safe and adequate (based on the fact that this is a typical American intake and deficiencies are extremely rare).

In the late 1980s, manganese made front page news in the popular press when it was reported that Bill Walton, then a professional basketball player, had a problem with his legs. A chemist analyzed Walton's blood and found a deficiency of manganese. The chemist went on to state that this deficiency was causing the bones of the legs to weaken and that the root of the problem was Walton's vegetarian diet. The chemist then stated that animal flesh was the only reliable source of manganese.

Although one of the functions of manganese is involved with the growth of bony tissues, the flaws in this story were several:

1. The richest sources of manganese are whole grains, legumes, nuts, and tea. Fruits and vegetables are moderate sources. Animal tissues, seafood, and dairy products are poor sources.[16]
2. Walton was not a vegetarian anyway. He consumed a macrobiotic diet and ate fish regularly.
3. Walton's great basketball prowess was attributed to the fact that he grew approximately five inches in less than two years when he was in high school. (Thus, he had the coordination of a medium-sized person in a very tall person's body.) Growth like this would likely not take place in the absence of manganese. (Although, from a purely speculative standpoint, this growth spurt may have depleted his manganese [and probably several other mineral] stores.)

In any event, attributing his problems to his (supposed) diet was unfortunate. No rebuttal was ever printed.

CHROMIUM

Chromium (Cr) is believed to assist the cells of the body in recognizing instructions from insulin to take in glucose. A large molecule called glucose tolerance factor (GTF) contains chromium (along with the B-vitamin niacin) in its biologically active form. At one time, the possibility that GTF would be classified as a vitamin was discussed, but because the body can manufacture GTF from its components, it does not qualify as a true vitamin.

The ESADDI is 50–200 mcg for adults. The current intake is estimated at 25–40 mcg daily, and this could explain why impaired glucose tolerance is so common. It is interesting that people deficient in chromium may exhibit either high or low blood glucose (hyper- or hypoglycemia). Chromium corrects both conditions, just as fiber slows absorption of sugars and similarly helps alleviate both.

Good sources of chromium include potatoes, brewer's yeast, molasses, whole grains, fruits, and vegetables. Refined carbohydrates (white flour, white sugar, etc.) have little or no chromium left, making it doubly difficult for the glucose in them to be regulated properly once absorbed.

SELENIUM (Se)

Selenium has received much good publicity since it was discovered that it functions as a part of the enzyme glutathione peroxidase, which is a potent antioxidant (similar in function to vitamin E) and thus anticarcinogenic. An RDA was first established for selenium in 1989. Like many other trace minerals, the content of selenium in foods is dependent on the soil in which it is grown. Probably for this reason, the richest source is considered to be Brazil nuts, because they are grown in the Amazon rainforest. Whole grains are also good sources. Molasses is a good source, since sugar cane is grown in deep, rich muck soil. The regular table sugar that is refined from it, however, has no trace minerals.

MOLYBDENUM (Mo)

Not much is heard about this mineral because it is widespread in common foods, including whole grains, dark green leafy vegetables, and legumes. One of its functions in the body is to help degrade sulfur-containing compounds, including the sulfur-containing amino acids methionine and cysteine and sulfites. The latter are often added as preservatives to foods, such as pre-cut lettuce served in some restaurants. Several people with asthma have had severe reactions to these sulfites, but it is still not clear whether or not this relates to their Mo status.

FLUORIDE (F)

A final entry for our list of nutrients that are added to our food supply by governmental fortification efforts (like vitamin D in milk and iodine in salt) is fluoride, often added to drinking water. Like chlorine, fluorine is a deadly gas, but fluoride, the ionic form of this element, is a constituent of bones and teeth and is considered an essential nutrient. Populations that live in areas where water naturally contains higher levels of fluoride have been found to have lower incidences of dental caries (cavities in their teeth). A theory that fluoride might make bones more resistant to osteoporosis has failed to be proved.

Fluoride has been added, in a concentration of one part per million, to many American public water supplies since 1945 in an attempt to reduce the incidence of dental cavities. This equates to 1 mg per liter. Thus, 8 cups of water, a typical daily adult intake, contains approximately 2 mg. The ESADDI is 1.5–4.0 mg. People who sweat profusely at work or play (physical laborers, athletes, etc.) may drink 16 cups of water daily, providing 4 mg of fluoride. Toxic doses can cause discoloration, or mottling, of the teeth. This condition, referred to as fluorosis, makes the teeth very strong but not very pretty. Some people object to public water fluoridation for this reason and also because of a still unproven theory that links excess fluoride to cancer. In any event, it is probably true that the people at whom the fluoride fortification is aimed (children, who are much more prone to caries than adults) do not drink very much water. They instead consume lots of soft drinks, which may or may not have been prepared with fluoridated water.

COBALT (Co)

Since its only known function is as a part of vitamin B-12 (cobalamin), cobalt is often not considered separately as a trace mineral. Unlike the chromium/GTF situation, the human body cannot manufacture cobalamin from cobalt. However, many microorganisms can, and some of them live in the human digestive tract. It is not clear just how much B-12 we can absorb from these organisms living inside us. Some have theorized that vegans benefit from them much more than others, possibly because of a more hospitable digestive tract.

In any event, cobalt must be present for B-12 to be produced anywhere; thus, the cobalt content of soil, if not our diet, ought to be paid some attention. Again, a plus for organic agriculture: it is well documented that vegans in poorer countries like Pakistan have much higher B-12 levels than those in richer countries. Though this is usually credited to higher microorganism contents in the drinking water, it is also possible that the organic farming methods (used out of necessity in poor countries) puts a lot more cobalt back in the soil.

NOTES

[13] A. Ascherio et al., "Dietary iron intake and risk of coronary disease among men," *Circulation* 89 (March 1994): 969–974.

[14] Paul Knekt et al., "Body iron stores and risk of cancer," *International Journal of Cancer* 56, no. 3 (February 1994) 379-382, DOI: 10.1002/ijc.2910560315.

[15] Melodie Anne Coffman, "Iron and Cancer," *LiveStrong*, June 18, 2011, http://www.livestrong.com/article/473732-iron-cancer/.

[16] L. Kathleen Mahan and Marian Arlin, *Krause's Food, Nutrition & Diet Therapy* (St. Louis, MO: Saunders, 1992), 135.

Practice Test: UNIT 12 — Trace Minerals

Study the **Information Summary** *and then try to complete this test from memory.**

1. Why do vegetarians who eat dairy products and eggs often become anemic?

2. How would you respond to someone who states that vegetarians may become anemic because they have no heme iron in their diet?

3. What is goiter, and how is it caused?

4. List the three sources contributing to overconsumption of iodine in the United States.

    i.

    ii.

    iii

5. How can the problem of phytates binding zinc in whole grains be overcome?

6. What component of cow's milk is an avid binder of zinc, and what is it (CHO, lipid, protein, vitamin, etc.)?

Practice Test: UNIT 12 — Trace Minerals

7. Why has high-dose supplementation with zinc been proved not to be a good idea?

8. Why might some people object to fluoridation of public drinking water?

9. How do you respond to someone who believes everyone should take supplements because the soils are depleted of nutrients?

10–14. Match the following with their principal known functions:

_____ 10. Chromium   a. Helps degrade sulfur-containing compounds

_____ 11. Cobalt   b. A part of vitamin B-12

_____ 12. Selenium   c. Needed for growth of bone

_____ 13. Manganese   d. Antioxidant

_____ 14. Molybdenum   e. Helps with glucose tolerance

*Answer Keys *begin on page 134.*

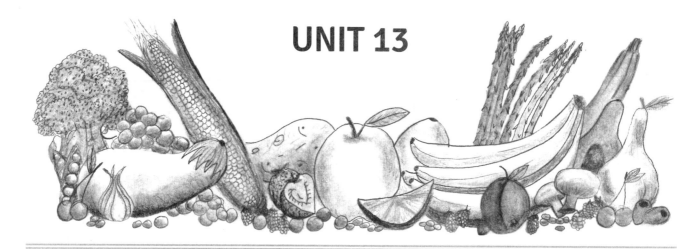

UNIT 13

Vegan Foods I

Information Summary

Foods are those substances that provide nutrition to the human body. There are thousands of such substances consumed throughout the world. The greatest variety of these comes from the plant kingdom. The next two chapters will look at some of these and also at the subject of evaluating foods in general.

It is recommended (though not required) that the student have access to a table of nutritional content of foods, usually found in the appendix of any nutrition textbook. (*Understanding Nutrition* by Ellie Whitney and Sharon Rady Rolfes provides one that is better than most because it contains analyses of several prepared vegetarian foods that other texts lack.) An inexpensive source is the United States government publication USDA Home and Garden Bulletin Number 72, *Nutritive Value of Foods*.

RATING FOODS

When discussing foods, there is a tendency to want to rate them, or at least rank them, as good or bad or somewhere in between. As you now should be aware, this is a complicated task. One could look at their total calorie content, their content of the various essential nutrients, their balance of energy nutrients (CHO–Fat–Protein), or their (lack of) content of undesirable constituents (cholesterol, saturated fats, environmental contaminants, etc.).

CALORIC DENSITY

One of the first questions people ask about a food is, "Is it fattening?" Of course, anything that contains any calories at all is fattening if you eat enough of it. What the questioner really wants to know is how many calories there are in a typical serving. The problem lies in defining a typical serving.

The term "caloric density" refers to the amount of calories in a food per given unit of weight or volume. Weight is a more exact and often more convenient measure (at least for someone with a good scale) than volume, given the consistency and shape of many foods. Consider, for instance, how the actual amount in a cup of cooked rice may vary depending on whether it is allowed to remain fluffy or is packed down hard or how difficult it is to measure the volume of a baked potato or a slice of tomato. Thus, the common measure of caloric density is calories/gram. Since a typical serving of many foods is approximately one-fourth pound (4 oz), many nutrient tables consider the nice round number of 100 grams (actually closer to 3.5 oz) as a serving size.

NUTRIENT DENSITY

Combining caloric density with the content of any essential nutrient in a food yields its nutrient density with respect to that nutrient. One nutrient at a time is examined, and a food is judged to be either a good or poor source of that nutrient. This is sometimes done per typical serving as eaten in this country or, on a more equitable basis, nutrients per calorie. Calories are the "currency" of diet; consuming more than a determined maximum amount of calories each day presents us with the risk of becoming overweight. Nutrient density is most often expressed as the amount of the nutrient per 100 kcals of food. Many health professionals do not like to use this measurement because some foods, especially many vegetables, are low in caloric density; a 100 kcal portion is considered large. Additionally, other foods, such as meats and full-fat dairy products, have such a high caloric density that a 100 kcal portion seems paltry. Raw leafy vegetables such as spinach and lettuce have approximately 10 kcal per cup; cooked vegetables often have only 40 kcal per cup. The nutrient density of these vegetables with respect to almost all essential nutrients is thus high, but dietitians contend that most people are not likely to eat large portions. On the other hand, a 3 oz hamburger patty (smaller than a "quarter-pounder") has approximately 240 kcal; a cup of ice cream has approximately 270 kcal. This concept is key to understanding what is meant by "important" nutrient sources, as discussed in the following section.

"IMPORTANT" VS. "GOOD" SOURCES OF NUTRIENTS

One statement often heard in nutrition circles is, "Food X (or food group Z) is an *important* source of nutrient Q." This is often heard in regard to calcium, riboflavin, and vitamin D; protein for milk (or dairy products); and iron and protein for meat. What this means is that given the current diet of a country such as the United States, a significant amount of nutrient Q is obtained from that food or group of foods. It does not mean that those foods are the best or the only *good* sources of that nutrient, and it does not even mean that those foods are a particularly rich source on a *per calorie basis* (nutrient density). What it does mean is that enough of those foods are consumed such that a relatively large amount of the nutrient gets consumed along with it. Even if the foods have a high nutrient density, it seems appropriate that before anyone refers to them as anything like a *good* source of a nutrient, account should be taken of other factors, such as environmental contaminants (much more prevalent in animal products than in plants because of the food chain hierarchy), cholesterol, saturated fat, etc. Even constituents such as protein, pre-formed vitamin A and/or vitamin D, and *concentrated* fiber (because of its tendency to hinder absorption) ought to be considered.

ENERGY NUTRIENT BALANCE

Another dimension that can be used for rating foods is the balance of energy nutrients. Remember that ideal human diets generally derive approximately 80% of their calories from carbohydrates, approximately 10% from fats, and approximately 10% from protein. Actually, the generous United States RDA for protein sets it at only 8% of calories, and the essential fatty acids are easily obtained at 9% of calories as fat. The numerical balance of 80/10/10 is easy to remember and work with and should be used as a guide, not as an absolute. Any food that deviates greatly from this pattern, however, may be considered unbalanced. This is not to say that such a food should not be eaten at all, but it becomes important to note how many total calories are consumed from that food. Of course, another food (or combination of foods) that is unbalanced in an opposite direction can offset it.

THE ENERGY NUTRIENT BALANCE OF ANIMAL PRODUCTS

It may be helpful here, for a point of comparison, to look at the approximate energy nutrient balance (ENB) of animal products. Except for milk with its lactose, all animal products have basically zero carbohydrates. Regular milk is approximately 25/50/25. Some people are fooled when they read the fat content of regular milk as being 3.5% butterfat. This refers to percentage by volume, which of course is largely water. It is not the percentage of calories from fat. Thus, "2%" milk has approximately half its fat removed, so the ratios become 35/30/35, while true skim milk has all its fat gone and so is 50/0/50.

Eggs are approximately 0/70/30. All of the fat is in the yolk, so when whites only are used, they contribute 0/0/100.

Most meats, such as beef and pork, are 0/70/30; the "lean" cuts, including "veal," are still approximately 0/55/45. Poultry flesh (skin removed prior to cooking) is approximately 0/30/70, while most nonfatty fish flesh is approximately 0/10/90.

It should be obvious that any diet built around these foods or any combination thereof will be excessive in fat or protein or both. It is little wonder that many people crave sweets (ENB of white sugar is 100/0/0) in an attempt to bring about balance. Usually all that is achieved is obesity and tooth decay.

UNDESIRABLE CONSTITUENTS IN FOODS

Another way to rate foods is their lack of undesirable constituents. As an example, you are already aware that cholesterol is only found in animal products. What many people do not realize is that the meat of any animal—cow, pig, chicken, turkey, or fish—has approximately the same amount of cholesterol. In this regard they are all about equal, and only those animal foods with all their fat removed (nonfat milk, egg whites) would rank higher. Of course, these latter items would rank much worse in regard to excess protein.

Where all animal products rank poorly is in regard to environmental contamination. Although much has been written in recent years about pesticide use on fruits and vegetables, remember that, because animals are higher in the food chain than plants, their flesh (and milk and eggs) will contain many times the concentration of pollutants. In fact, one of the factors that led to the banning of the use of the pesticide DDT in the United States several decades ago was a study that showed that the breast milk of women was exceeding the level allowable for public sale in cow's milk. Why would human beings have more of this toxic pesticide in their systems than cows? The answer is because most of us eat an animal product–based diet, while cows eat a plant-based diet. To prove the point, the breast milk of human vegetarian women was analyzed and found to contain low DDT levels. Of course, rather than recommend that we all become vegetarian, the government banned the use of the pesticide. Incidentally, only the *use* of DDT was banned, not its manufacture. American companies continue to make it and then sell it to other countries, such as Mexico, where it is used on crops. Much of this produce is then exported back to the United States—another reason (besides compassion for the hungry) not to buy foods from poor countries.

The refined sugar content of foods is often used to rank breakfast cereals. Since sugars are a natural part of the plant foods, it is advisable (rather than avoiding them altogether) to keep sugars to an appropriate level in relation to the fiber and other natural constituents present.

FOOD GROUPS & FOOD GUIDES

How to group foods in order to create simple food guides for teaching purposes continues to be a difficult task for nutrition educators. Beginning a few decades ago, the United States government issued promotional materials about the twelve food groups. They subsequently reduced it to seven, then five, and finally to the infamous four food groups many of us were exposed to in the second grade. Thankfully, and over the objections of the food industry's special interest groups, these groups were re-formed into a pyramid that no longer gave animal-derived foods equal status with plant foods. The four food groups implied that half the foods we eat should come from animals (two out of four groups: meats and dairy). Our epidemic of diet-related disease can be easily attributed to this faulty notion.

Why did anyone ever create that system? The rationale for having a dairy group was as a source of calcium and riboflavin. The meat group was to provide protein and iron. As you are now aware, all of these can easily be obtained from plant-derived foods. The sole rationale one could pose for including animal products is B-12, and so vegan food guides usually include a footnote to include a source of it (either fortified foods or a periodic supplement) to allay those fears. It is certainly a small price to pay to avoid excess calories, saturated fats, cholesterol, and excess protein. Unfortunately, the imprint of the four food groups will for a while haunt older textbooks and the minds of people educated in nutrition before the 1990s.

It is important to remember that no grouping of foods was ever handed to us by Mother Nature; they were fabrications based partially on the "best" of what was commonly eaten but mostly on what governmental agencies such as the United States Department of Agriculture (USDA) wanted to promote for sale. The USDA was created to help American farmers sell their products. Its role as an advocate of good nutrition is secondary.

FOOD EXCHANGE SYSTEMS

Ever since the advent of insulin treatments for people with diabetes, measuring the amount of carbohydrates in a person's diet has become critical. It has to correspond closely to the amount of insulin being administered each day. Too much CHO would cause the blood sugar to stay elevated; too little CHO would cause a reaction known as insulin shock, in which the blood sugar falls critically low.

Thus, a system of food categories was developed according to the CHO content and put into lists called exchanges. The patient could then be instructed to choose so many exchanges from each of several groups each day, and the dietitian would be assured that the CHO content would remain constant.

Weight-reduction diets are sometimes based on these exchanges because they are an easy way to control total calorie intake, since each exchange should contain a constant amount of fat and protein as well. For instance, one fruit exchange may be one apple, one-half of a banana, or one-fourth cup of grape juice, since each contains approximately 10 g of CHO and thus 40 kcal. One bread exchange is one slice of bread or one-half cup of pasta, since both contain approximately 15 g CHO and approximately 2 g protein (total approximately 70 kcal). One of the obvious problems with the traditional exchange system was that it ignored fiber, now known to have an important role in regulating blood sugar and obesity.

GROUPING VEGAN FOODS

Foods from plants can be grouped into the following categories: fruits, vegetables, grains, beans, nuts, and seeds. These should not be viewed as groups in the sense of having to eat from each one every day (or ever). There is no food or group of foods that is necessary for human health. These groupings simply categorize foods with similar qualities and/or origins. There may seem to be overlap between groups because some foods are versatile. Corn, for instance, is sometimes used as a vegetable and sometimes as a grain. Additional confusion may be caused because some of these have botanical definitions (fruit) while others (vegetables) are principally culinary terms.

FRUITS

The original usage of the word "fruit" implied "any plant-derived food" (hence, the expression *fruits of the earth*). In the eighteenth century, the science of botany altered the definition to mean the fleshy material surrounding seeds of any plant, edible or not. In the food terminology of today, we refer to the edible sweet and/or sour flesh surrounding seeds plus a few other sweet and/or sour parts of certain plants as "fruits." Strawberries, which we will consider as berries, are not a true fruit at all but are actually a part of the flower. The tiny seeds on them have a thin coating around each one that is technically the fruit. Rhubarb is also considered a fruit even though it is only the stem of the plant that is eaten. Those fruits that have a more bland taste, such as tomatoes, cucumbers, squash, and eggplant, are considered vegetables. Avocados are considered fruits by some people (they are sometimes called "alligator pears"), but because they are more often eaten in vegetable salads than fruit salads, they will be discussed as a vegetable.

Categories of common fruits eaten in North America are citrus, berries (including grapes), pome fruits (apples, pears), stone fruits (plums, cherries, peaches, nectarines, apricots), melons (which are actually in the squash family), and other fruits such as bananas (botanically they are berries), figs, dates, rhubarb, and kiwifruit. The energy nutrient ratio (CHO–Fat–Protein) of most fruits is approximately 90–5–5. Theoretically, an all-fruit diet could be marginally low in protein and fat. Some berries do have slightly higher protein content, presumably because the seeds are eaten. Digestibility of this protein may be questioned (consider how these seeds tend to "go right through") unless care is taken to chew finely. The nutrient most people associate with fruits is ascorbic acid. It is abundant not only in citrus fruits but in some berries (strawberries and raspberries have a lot; blueberries and grapes don't have much), melons (cantaloupe is especially rich), and kiwifruit. The pome and stone fruits don't have much ascorbic acid, nor do bananas, dates, figs, or rhubarb. It is ironic that fruits such as apples, pears, and peaches are not abundant in ascorbic acid, although they are all in the rose family. The fruits of the wild rose, which are small berries often called rose hips, are a rich source of ascorbic acid. Though many people feel confident getting their vitamin C from their morning orange juice, it is not well publicized that orange juice has less than one-fourth the nutrient density of vitamin C that occurs in whole oranges. Some is left behind in the pulp, and much is lost on exposure to air. Vitamin A as beta-carotene is a bright yellow-orange pigment; fruits of that coloring (cantaloupe, apricots, peaches, tangerines) are rich sources. Paler-colored fruits (white grapefruit, bananas, honeydew melon, pineapple) have little.

VEGETABLES

The word "vegetable" originally meant any plant (hence, "Is it animal, vegetable, or mineral?"). In the eighteenth century, when botanists altered the meaning of fruit (see above), a word was needed to identify the nonfruit parts of plants that were eaten. Since most of these were eaten with the main part of the meal (rather than dessert) this remains as the distinction between the two, regardless of the part of the plant from which they are derived. What we call vegetables today may be roots or tubers (carrots, potatoes), stems (celery, asparagus), fruits (cucumbers, tomatoes), leaves (lettuce, spinach), or whole plants (mushrooms, sprouts). Because of the variation in the parts of plants represented, there is more variation in their nutritional makeup than in fruits. The CHO–Fat–Protein balance of most vegetables is approximately 65/10/25. This seems high in protein, and it is, but most vegetables are so low in total calories that they do not have the power to imbalance a total day's intake significantly. An exception is the mature legumes (beans, peas) discussed separately in the next chapter. The calorie-dense, starchy root and tuber vegetables, such as potatoes, have an energy nutrient balance closer to that of the grains, in the area of 80/10/10. Anyone who worries that they may be getting too much protein from vegetables need only balance them with fruits. Avocados are an anomaly in terms of their high fat content (olives are similar, but because they are only eaten as a condiment, they are included in the next chapter). The energy nutrient balance of Florida avocados is approximately 25/70/5; the California varieties are even richer at 13/82/5. This is one food to use sparingly if a low-fat diet is desired. Like fruits, many vegetables are good sources of vitamin C, especially leafy greens and tomatoes. Since heat breaks down ascorbic acid, cooking time must be considered. (Published tables of nutritional content of foods assume *minimum* cooking times.) Also, like fruits, color is a clue to vitamin A (beta-carotene) content. As expected, carrots, sweet potatoes, and winter squash are rich sources. Pale-colored ones (cauliflower, summer squash) are not as good or are downright poor. What may be deceptive, however, are two facts. First, dark green vegetables such as broccoli and spinach are excellent sources. The chlorophyll in them masks the color of beta-carotene. The second misleading fact is that there are other pigments, especially red ones such as betacyanin in beets, that might lead one to believe beta-carotene is present when actually it is not in any great amount. Beets are low in vitamin A activity (a mere 4 RE per 100 kcal), but beet greens, often used as a vegetable separately, are loaded with beta-carotene (1,835 RE per 100 kcal; USRDA = 1,000 RE).

Practice Test: UNIT 13 — Vegan Foods I

Study the **Information Summary** *and then try to complete this test from memory.* *

1. How would you respond to someone who says that vegans have an unbalanced diet because they don't eat from all of the "food groups"?

2. How does "caloric density" differ from "nutrient density"?

3. List five categories of fruits commonly eaten, giving at least one example of each, and note which categories are generally good sources of vitamin C.

    i.

    ii.

    iii.

    iv.

    v.

4. How do potatoes and avocados differ from most other vegetables in terms of energy nutrient balance?

5. How does the energy nutrient balance of fruits compare with that of most vegetables? How can they be used together to "balance" a day's diet?

6. In what way is color a clue to the vitamin A content of a fruit or vegetable? How can color be misleading in this regard?

7. What advantage do vegan foods have over animal products in regard to environmental contaminants? How was this demonstrated in regard to DDT?

Answer Keys begin on page 134.

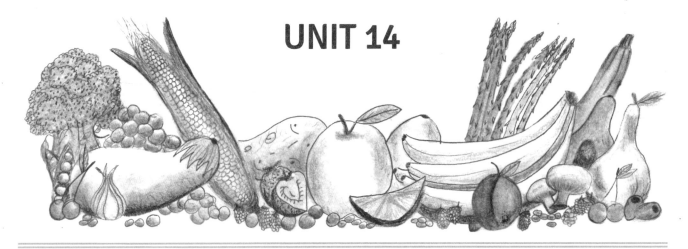

UNIT 14

Vegan Foods II

Information Summary

Discussed in this chapter are: grains, beans, nuts and seeds, condiments, and animal-product substitutes.

GRAINS

Grains, also called **cereals**, are the seeds of grasses. Although there are approximately 8,000 species of grass, only a few are commonly used as food by human beings: rice, wheat, rye, oats, barley, millet, and corn. Triticale, a cross between rye and wheat, is becoming increasingly popular, as are some grains used in pre-Columbian America, such as amaranth and quinoa (pronounced KEEN-wa). In general, grains have an energy nutrient balance (ENB) near the ideal of 80/10/10 (CHO-Fat-Protein). Oats have the highest fat content at 16%, still well within the limits of a low-fat diet.

The structure of any whole grain consists of four major parts:

1. An outer **bran** layer which contains most of the fiber
2. An **aluerone** layer just inside the bran, which contains a large amount of the water-soluble vitamins and the minerals

Figure 14.1 — Structure of a Grain

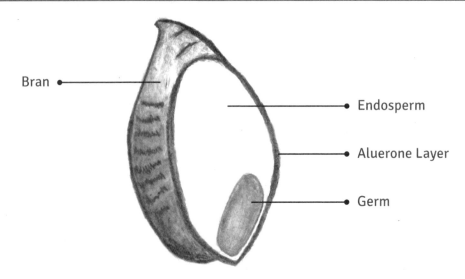

Bran

Endosperm

Aluerone Layer

Germ

3. The **germ**, which contains most of the lipid, along with the fat-soluble vitamins and a dispropor-tionate (relative to its small size) amount of protein

4. The **endosperm**, the largest part, which contains mostly starch and protein

GLUTEN

Grains contain several different proteins. One of them, gliadin (particularly abundant in wheat), is a part of the chemical complex called gluten that forms when ground-up grain (flour) is mixed with water. Gluten has great stretching ability and is the reason why breads can rise so much without crumbling. Gluten is also the basis for making seitan, a meat substitute. Gliadin, however, causes a reaction in some people, a condition known as gluten-sensitive enteropathy, or celiac sprue. It affects the intestinal lining and sometimes the skin. People with this condition must avoid wheat products, as well as rye and barley, which also contain gluten but in lesser amounts than wheat, which is why breads made solely from those grains don't rise as well. Oats potentially can be a problem due to cross-contamination, though a small number of people with celiac disease cannot seem to tolerate even uncontaminated oats very well. Corn and rice are gliadin-free and so are acceptable for people with this condition, but breads made from them crumble severely.

NUTRIENTS IN GRAINS

The most noted nutritional shortcoming of grains is that they have little vitamin C or vitamin A. Grains are good sources of the B vitamins (except B-12) and minerals, although mineral content will vary greatly depending on soil and farming methods. The germs of grains have adequate vitamin E to protect their polyunsaturated fatty acids and even have a little vitamin D as well.

GRAIN PRODUCTS

Breads are baked products made from grain flours that are usually combined with some source of leavening, often a living yeast called baker's yeast (not to be confused with nutritional yeast, which is a type of brewer's yeast that has been enriched with vitamin B-12 and other nutrients). The yeast-raising process seems to inactivate the mineral-binding phytates present in the bran layer. Breads leavened without yeast, such as those made with baking soda or powder, or those not leavened (flat breads) may have much less available mineral content. Refined grain products have no phytates present because the bran layer has been removed, but they don't have much mineral content left either, unless enriched (and usually the only mineral added back is iron).

When most people speak of bran, they are referring to wheat bran, which is almost pure fiber. Oat bran, as it is sold, usually has a significant part of the endosperm still attached and thus has some caloric value (approx-imately one-half of the caloric density of whole oats). This fact, along with the fact that it has much more soluble fiber, makes oat bran a better balanced "food," although still not ideal compared to whole grains.

Wheat germ is considered by many as a "health food," given its abundance of fat-soluble vitamins. It is a little too rich in its energy nutrient balance (50/25/25), and since its caloric density is high (400 kcal per 100 gm), overconsumption is easy.

Refined grains are generally all endosperm. Once the bran is milled off, the oils in the germ become exposed to the air and would turn rancid, so it is also removed. The aluerone layer is usually removed as well because it has a light brown color, and a pure white product is usually desired. Graham flour is refined wheat flour that has its aluerone layer left on. It was originated by Sylvester Graham, one of the pioneers of the vegetarian movement in the West, mostly remembered for the graham cracker, which is still made (though only partially) with his "better" flour.

Whole wheat flour, which contains germ, bran, aluerone, and endosperm, seems obviously the best choice, and it is, as far as choices of flour go. However, remember that when fiber is divided up too finely, such as in the flour grinding process, it loses much of its functional ability. It is better to consume whole grains or at least just cracked grains, which are whole grains that have been broken into coarse pieces. Many health-conscious bread manufacturers add some of one or both of these.

Although the word "cereal" is technically synonymous with grain, it is commonly used to refer only to those products eaten either hot or cold in a bowl for breakfast (or midnight snacks). There is tremendous variation in the nutritional content, some being fortified with vitamins and minerals to the extent that they are classified as a supplement rather than a food by the USDA. The closest products to simple whole grains are oatmeal and cracked whole wheat (common brand in the United States: Wheatena). Among the ready-to-eat varieties, the closest thing is shredded wheat, although it doesn't look like it (it tastes like it, though). The first ready-to-eat cereal, corn flakes, was originated by John Harvey Kellogg, a pioneer of American vegetarianism.

BEANS

Many people think that vegans must eat some beans every day to assure adequate protein. Hopefully you know by now that this is ridiculous, and bean-haters can feel free to become vegan. Anything that grows in a pod is called a **legume**. Most of these are what we commonly call beans and peas. Peanuts are also legumes, but their nutritional makeup (ENB: 12/70/18) more resembles other nuts; for that reason, they are discussed in that section below. Soybeans are unique among beans in their exceptionally high protein and fat content (ENB: 21/42/37). Most beans have approximately the same energy nutrient balance as vegetables at 70/5/25, but since they have more calories in a typical serving (higher caloric density), the high protein content has much more significance. In *The McDougall Plan*, John McDougall, MD, recommends that no more than the equivalent of one cup of cooked beans be included in the daily adult diet to avoid excess protein intake. Since this represents approximately 15 grams of protein and since all other whole foods eaten will contain some protein, it is pretty good advice.

Those beans that are in their pods before they are fully mature (such as green [string] beans, yellow wax beans, snow peas, etc.) have much lower caloric densities and so are more appropriately considered as vegetables. Green peas are intermediate in their caloric density.

BEAN PRODUCTS

Most bean products are made from soybeans; many of them are used as replacements for animal-derived foods. **Soy milk** is made by blending and then straining cooked soybeans. It is commonly used in infant formulas for those babies allergic to cow's milk. **Tofu**, or bean curd, is made from soy milk that has been coagulated with a chemical agent. Often, this agent is calcium sulfate, and the tofu made with it is a rich source of calcium (approximately 140 mg/100 kcal; compare to cottage cheese at 75 mg/100 kcal). Tofu, because it is made from soy milk that originally was strained, has little fiber. A point of caution about high-protein, low-fiber foods like tofu is that they are as prone to spoilage as milk products and should be refrigerated diligently. Many grocers, probably under pressure from dairy people, put tofu in their produce section rather than in the dairy case. The dairy lobby would like the public to consider it a "vegetable," not a dairy substitute. Unfortunately, produce is not as strictly refrigerated as dairy (because fruits and vegetables don't become spoiled nearly as quickly). Many people do not like tofu because all they have tasted is some that was poorly refrigerated and thus had developed an unpleasant aroma. When fresh, it has almost no aroma and tastes "milky," not "beany." Aseptically packaged tofu does not have to be refrigerated, and it retains its fresh flavor (more precisely, lack of strong flavor) longer. **Tempeh** is a fermented product made from whole soybeans, sometimes with a grain added. Unlike tofu, all the fiber of the bean is still intact. Up until the late 1980s, it was believed that all tempeh was a good source of vitamin B-12. The making of tempeh originated in Indonesia, where tempeh is still widely eaten. The way it is produced there allows some microorganisms that manufacture cobalamin to get into it. American manufacturers of it, however, are required to use much more antiseptic conditions, and the B-12-producing microorganisms tend to get excluded.

Miso is a fermented soybean paste (some types have a grain added) with a large amount of added salt. It is made from whole beans but is finely ground, so the fiber may be of less value. It contains approximately 600 mg of sodium per tablespoon. It is mainly used as a base for soups, gravies, and salad dressings. **Soy sauce** is a liquid extract of salted, fermented soybeans and sometimes wheat. It contains approximately 1000 mg of sodium per tablespoon—quite a lot, but still much less than pure salt (6,000 mg Na per tablespoon). Aging of soy sauce develops its flavor. A small amount can add more taste to a dish without having to use too much. **Tamari** refers to aged soy sauce with no wheat added. **Shoyu** is aged soy sauce with wheat added. Most commercial soy sauce sold in supermarkets in North America is not aged; it instead has coloring and flavorings added. There are reduced-sodium soy sauces now available, but they usually have preservatives added to replace the preserving power of the salt. **Hummus** is a Middle Eastern dish made from mashed garbanzo beans, which is one of the richer beans (ENB: 65/13/22) though much less so than soy. Hummus is made by mashing these and adding tahini, a sesame seed paste. This thickener makes the dish fairly high in fat (ENB: 46/43/11).

NUTS & SEEDS

Another myth about protein in vegan diets (besides the one that we must eat beans every day to get it) is that nuts are abundant in it. Nonvegans often declare, "Where do you get your protein...from nuts?" It is possible that people like asking that because it gives them the opportunity to use the word that in their minds describes vegans in general.

The term "nuts" technically refers to the high-fat seed coatings of certain trees. As mentioned above, peanuts—a legume—are included in this category of foods because of their high fat content. The average ENB of nuts is approximately 15/75/10. The 10% protein figure is what usually surprises people. The only truly low-fat nuts are chestnuts (ENB: 87/8/5). Although most nuts are laden with fat, they do have plenty of fiber, and their fat is mostly unsaturated. As long as nuts are in their shells, oxygen cannot get to the fats and they do not turn rancid. The only nuts that are high in saturated fatty acids are coconuts.

By far the most common form in which nuts are eaten in North America is peanut butter. It is sometimes sold in its natural state (ground-up peanuts, with or without added salt), but most commercial peanut butters have hydrogenated fats added to them (some of the unsaturated peanut oil is removed) to keep them from separating and to maintain freshness longer. Natural peanut butter needs to be stirred and then refrigerated.

Various other seeds are consumed like nuts: sunflower, sesame, pumpkin, poppy, etc. They are similar in fat content to most nuts. Tahini (mentioned above as an ingredient in garbanzo bean–based hummus) is to sesame seeds what peanut butter is to peanuts. It makes a tasty base for salad dressings and gravies. It has the remarkable property of getting thicker when combined with an acidic liquid, such as lemon juice or vinegar, and then water.

CONDIMENTS

Olives are the fattiest things that grow on plants. Their ENB of 7/91/3 is abominable. Yet because they are rich in fiber, and because their fat is mostly monounsaturated (the least of all evils, fat-wise), and because they are usually just eaten as pickled condiments (in their raw state they are unbearably bitter), nature can be forgiven. They have less potential to be fattening than nuts because their higher water content makes them much less calorie dense (115 kcal/100 g vs. approximately 550 kcal/100 g for nuts). However, for sodium-sensitive people prone to hypertension, olives could be dangerous (approximately 100 mg Na per large green olive).

Other **pickles** (usually cucumbers or other vegetables) generally have equally high salt contents to condemn them, but otherwise they can be a low-fat, high-fiber snack. There has been some association noted between high consumption of pickled products and stomach cancer in Asia, where people eat such foods (including pickled and salt-cured meats and fish) frequently.

Sweets are products rich in simple carbohydrates and largely devoid of fiber. There are many sweeteners available, probably the most nutritious of which is **blackstrap molasses**, created early during the sugar (sucrose) refining process. It still contains no fiber, but it has significant amounts of several essential nutrients, including calcium (300 mg/100 kcal), iron (11 mg/100 kcal), and potassium (1300 mg/100kcal). It is ironic that such a rich source of nutrition is made available during the production of the notoriously empty calorie white sugar.

VEGAN POINT OF INFORMATION

Many people assume that to be vegan is to be "health conscious" and that such things as concentrated sweets are "not part of the diet." Naturally, this depends on one's motivation for being vegan, but part of this myth is perpetuated by the fact that many vegan purists refuse white sugar. Their reason for doing so is that a part of the refining process involves filtering the sugar through a column of animal-bone charcoal (purchased from slaughterhouses). None of the bone is supposed to get into the final product (the purpose of the filtering is to purify the sugar of other substances, not to add anything). Nonetheless, this indirect support of the slaughter industry makes some uncomfortable, and their diet certainly doesn't suffer from excluding purified sucrose.

ANIMAL PRODUCT SUBSTITUTES

Some vegans apparently miss the taste and/or texture of animal products or wish to find substitutes for them in nonvegan recipes. A few of the replacement possibilities are discussed here.

EGG SUBSTITUTES

One of the more difficult tasks for the vegan cook is the replacement of eggs in recipes that require their binding ability (cakes, casseroles, etc.). There are manufactured powders available (usually with a potato starch base), but some people object to the synthetic ingredients these seem to have. Some more "natural" substitutes that work fairly well are chickpea (garbanzo bean) flour, tofu, arrowroot starch, and, believe it or not, apricots blended in a little water. These, of course, will vary greatly in their nutritional content; it is fruitless (except for the apricots) to try to compare them to eggs since they will be just a minor part of the diet.

MEAT ANALOGUES

Products that resemble various meats have been made in Asia for centuries. Here in the West it has principally been the Seventh-day Adventists, a Christian sect that advocates a vegetarian diet, who have manufactured and consumed these. They are usually made from soy, wheat, and/or peanut proteins and sold either canned or frozen or as powdered mixes. Some have egg whites added as binders; others are purely vegan. Most are fortified with nutrients, including vitamin B-12, to approximate the nutrient density of meats. Many health-oriented people refuse these products because they are highly "processed," often containing isolated proteins. They also generally have high sodium contents and sometimes additives such as artificial colorings and flavorings.

MILK & MILKS

The definition of **milk** is "any oily substance held in suspension in a watery substance." Thus, any fat-containing food can be blended in liquid and used as a milk. The most common use of the term is to refer to the secretion from the mammary glands of female mammals. In the United States we assume any food substance containing milk is cow's milk. Elsewhere, however, goat and sheep milk are common, and horse's milk was historically used. What we have been experiencing over the last 40 years or so in North America, in regard to the promotion of cow's milk as a wonderful food for everyone, is a classic case of a food fad. A food fad is a prevalent feeling that one must consume a particular product in order to maintain health. The only perfectly complete food for infant human beings is human milk. For children and adults, no one food is "perfect" and certainly not cow's milk. The fact that over half of the human beings in the world become lactose intolerant by the age of three should be proof enough.

Compared to human milk, cow's milk has a much higher mineral (especially sodium) and protein content, both of which put a strain on an infant's kidneys to excrete excesses. The protein in cow's milk is also allergenic to many human beings, and for this reason, soy milk–based infant formulas are now used more commonly than cow milk–based ones. Thus, even for infants the notion that (cow's) milk is somehow "nature's most perfect food" has fallen short.

Commercially available vegan milks are made from soy, rice, almond, coconut, and a number of other sources. Vegan milk can also be easily prepared at home from any grain, nut, or seed, all of which may have their fiber intact. Milks made from grains (usually these are cooked first, although uncooked rolled oats do fine) will have a lower fat content than those made from nuts and seeds. For vegan milks to duplicate the texture and taste of cow's milk, the following three steps must take place:

1. All fiber needs to be strained out.

2. Salt must be added (cow's milk has approximately 80 mg Na/100 kcal; grains, nuts and seeds have approximately 2 mg/100 kcal).

3. A small amount of sweetener (since cow's milk has a lot of lactose to make it taste slightly sweet) needs to be added.

None of these modifications are positive ones nutritionally, of course, but still may be a worthwhile trade-off to avoid cholesterol, saturated fats, and environmental contaminants. The question of calcium (and sometimes riboflavin) is often brought up when milk replacements are mentioned. The amounts in these vegan milks will depend on what particularly they are made from (and even how they were originally grown: organically grown grains from Asia have been found to have several hundred times the calcium content of commercially available ones here) and how they are processed. A less complicated and more reasonable approach to assuring adequate intake of these nutrients is to get them from consistently rich sources like leafy greens and not make any milk a disproportionate part of the diet.

FOOD SAFETY

By far most cases of **food poisoning** (sickness caused by eating food contaminated with disease-causing organisms) are from animal products. However, some plant-derived foods can harbor pathogenic microorganisms, especially those foods that have been processed (such as tofu). For this reason, it is wise to treat all moist, processed foods the same (dried foods don't provide enough water for microbes to grow much): don't eat them if they have been allowed to stand at a temperature between 40° and 140° F (equivalent to approximately 4° C and 60° C) for more than two hours. Thus, 40° F is considered safe refrigeration temperature, and 140° F is considered safe heat-storage temperature. (There are other preservation methods, of course, such as salting and pickling, that prevent microbe growth).

Practice Test: UNIT 14 — Vegan Foods II

Study the **Information Summary** *and then try to complete this test from memory.**

1–7. Match the category of food with its approximate energy nutrient balance (% calories from CHO–Fat–Protein).

(Selections may be used more than once.)

_____ 1. Olives a. 90/5/5

_____ 2. Green vegetables b. 80/10/10

_____ 3. Fruits c. 70/5/25

_____ 4. Grains d. 15/75/10

_____ 5. Beans (other than soybeans) e. 7/90/3

_____ 6. Nuts (except chestnuts) f. 65/10/25

_____ 7. Avocados

8–11. Match the grain product with its main nutritional drawback:

_____ 8. Wheat germ a. concentrated fiber

_____ 9. Whole wheat fiber b. concentrated fat and protein

_____ 10. Enriched white flour c. fiber too finely divided

_____ 11. Bran d. fiber deficient

12. How do soybeans differ from other beans?

13. What are tofu and tempeh, and what is different about their composition in terms of nutrition?

14. Why are peanuts more properly treated as nuts rather than as legumes (which they are botanically)?

Practice Test: UNIT 14 — Vegan Foods II

15. How do most commercial peanut butters differ from natural peanut butter?

16. What is the chemical definition of "milk"?

17. List three nutritional advantages for human adult use of a grain milk rather than cow milk. (Hints: fiber, fat, sodium)

    i.

    ii

    iii.

18. List three vegan substitutes for eggs in recipes.

    i.

    ii

    iii.

19. The safe holding temperature for prepared foods is below _____ F or above _____ F.

*Answer Keys *begin on page 134.*

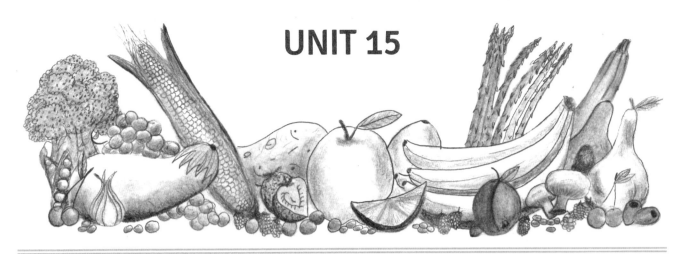

UNIT 15

Diet-Related Chronic Disease I

POINT OF MEDICAL INFORMATION

One must always be cautious to distinguish between using diet to reduce one's risk of getting a disease, or at least of getting it prematurely, and claiming that diet can cure or even treat any disease. The only diseases for which nutrition has proved to be a cure are those accurately diagnosed as frank nutrient deficiencies (and even for those, only licensed medical practitioners are permitted to make the diagnosis and prescribe the treatment). Diet therapy, which dietitians are trained in, is an adjunct to medical treatment, often done merely to support the patient in adequate nutriture. This and the following unit are not designed to be a course in diet therapy, nor are they intended to be used as any guide to treatment for any condition. They are a discussion of common disorders and some of the studies that revealed their possible connections to one or more elements of diet.

The science of nutrition was originally framed around preventing the occurrence of acute deficiency disease conditions like beriberi, scurvy, and pellagra. Its success in that regard is evident in that these are extremely rare in modern societies today. What are common, and actually the leading causes of death in North America, are conditions such as cardiovascular disease (which causes heart attacks and strokes), high blood pressure, diabetes, osteoporosis, etc. These diseases are termed chronic because they can be present for long periods of time before consequences become serious. It seems likely that their causes are chronic as well (diet, smoking, lack of exercise, etc.).

Relating diseases other than acute nutrient deficiencies to diet is a difficult task in the eyes of pure science, however. There are many other lifestyle and environmental factors that accompany differences in diet. Since diet is particular to each species, experiments using nonhuman animals have little use in defining the ideal human diet. The only good experiments that could prove a connection between these conditions and diet are long-term ones with human subjects, many of whom would be expected to die prematurely (not easy to find volunteers for those). Yet over the last few decades, many studies have demonstrated that diet is an important, and possibly the most important, cause of several chronic diseases.

CARDIOVASCULAR DISEASE

Ischemia is the medical term for any situation in which blood flow is cut off to any tissue due to blockage or constriction of the supplying blood vessel. Lack of oxygen results, which causes death of tissue (necrosis).

If this gets extensive enough to compromise the function of the area it is called an **infarct**.

The blood vessels that surround the heart and provide oxygen to its musculature (the **myocardium**) are called **coronary** arteries (because they resemble a crown over the heart). When any of these arteries or arterioles (small arteries) becomes blocked, a **myocardial infarction** (MI) can result. By far the most common cause of a blockage here is **atherosclerotic plaque** buildup, a yellowish substance that resembles oatmeal but is composed mainly of cholesterol. When the plaque is in the smaller vessels, the disease is called **arteriosclerosis**; when in the larger or medium-sized vessels, it is just called **atherosclerosis**.

Coronary heart disease (CHD) is any disease involving the coronary blood flow, but by far the largest proportion of people with this disease has atherosclerotic plaque causing the trouble. Buildup of plaque can also contribute to development of higher-than-normal blood pressure (**hypertension**). As vessels become smaller, the blood has to be pumped at a higher pressure to get it around the body. Hypertension is generally without symptoms until something ruptures. When this rupture occurs in a vessel leading to the brain, the result is called a **stroke**.

Animal protein—not just animal fat—intake has been directly linked to increased risk of heart disease.[17] CHD and stroke are the first and third leading causes of death, respectively, in the United States.

A landmark study that identified elevated blood cholesterol as a risk factor for CHD was the Framingham Heart Study begun in 1949 under the direction of Dr. William Castelli. More than 5,000 adults between the ages of 30 and 62 were chosen from this Massachusetts town and given health checkups for the remainder of their lives. (Approximately half were still alive as of 1985.) Later studies have shown how dietary factors such as dietary cholesterol, saturated fats, and animal protein as well as nondietary factors (cigarette smoking, lack of exercise) also influence blood cholesterol.[18]

Some short-term studies (often those with biased sponsorship) have reported dissimilar results. One faulty approach that has been taken is assuming that any slight improvement in diet (for instance, lowering fat intake from 40% of calories to 30%) ought to have measurable benefit. It often doesn't, and then the conclusion is drawn that fat is not the culprit. This all-too-moderate approach may be done because some worry that a diet below 30% of calories as fat may be undesirable because it can lower HDL-cholesterol (the "good" kind). Having a high HDL-cholesterol level is protective if overall cholesterol is high. If total cholesterol is low, however, it has no apparent effect on disease risk.

HYPERTENSION

Many different conditions can cause elevation of one's blood pressure. Essential hypertension is the term used for elevated blood pressure that cannot be attributed to any other health problem. It may be contributed to by buildup of atherosclerotic plaque (see above), but many people have plaque buildup and yet don't have a very elevated blood pressure. Excess sodium intake contributes to hypertension in some people; in others, excess body weight (obesity) is a major factor (though not all obese people have hypertension). Blood pressure is measured according to the height (in millimeters) of a mercury (Hg) column it can support. Two numbers are given: the systolic pressure, which relates to the volume of blood pumped with each beat, and the diastolic pressure, which measures the resistance of the blood vessels to the flow. Usually the diastolic number is more significant: if it is over 90 mm Hg, hypertension is said to exist. Generally the systolic number is supposed to be under 140 mm Hg to be considered normal.

VEGAN POINT OF INFORMATION

Switching to a vegan diet generally lowers one's blood pressure approximately 10 mm Hg. No study (and many have been attempted) has been able to isolate the exact reason why. It has been theorized that the same stress hormones in meat extract that may cause superfluous stomach acid secretion might also cause blood pressure to rise. It is well known that stress increases blood pressure. Diets for people with hypertension classically are low in sodium, but this doesn't help much in many cases and almost never makes the condition disappear completely. A low-sodium diet is critical, however, for a different but sometimes related acute condition: congestive heart failure.

CONGESTIVE HEART FAILURE

When the heart gradually loses its capability for normal function (most frequently from complications of atherosclerosis), a set of bodily events occurs that culminates in a condition in which the kidneys are unable to excrete sodium adequately. This results in fluid retention (water stays behind with the salt) known as edema. All organ systems become congested with fluid, and the term "congestive heart failure" is applied.

The dietary therapy that accompanies medical treatment for this disorder is sodium restriction. Depending on the severity of the disease, this may be as liberal as merely dictating "no added salt" (in which as much as 4,000 mg of Na is allowed) or as limited as "severe sodium restriction" (in which only 250 mg of Na is permitted). Intermediate (and more common) levels are "mild restriction" (2,500 mg), "moderate restriction" (1,000 mg), and "strict restriction" (500 mg).

In any case, a mistaken impression people often have is that it was excess salt intake that caused the condition in the first place. Not true. This is similar to the mistaken impression about **diabetes mellitus** (see next unit), in which sugar is restricted, though it is not the cause of the disease. In both instances, fats are the culprit, and it is in coping with those fats that these conditions occur. The limitations on salt and sugar are necessary (at least temporarily) to delay further complications.

CANCER

Cancer is a class of disorders characterized by abnormal growth of cells. Collectively they are the second leading cause of death in the United States. The factors involved in cancer incidence are divided into two categories: initiators and promoters. Initiators are what we usually called carcinogens or those compounds capable of causing mutation in cells sufficient to bring the change approximately to a cancerous state. The putrefaction of animal protein in the colon, for instance, releases chemicals that are carcinogens, as does the charcoal broiling of flesh foods. The oxygenated free radicals of rancid fats are also carcinogens. Other carcinogens abound in the environment, but a well-functioning immune system has a great ability to negate their effects unless overwhelmed. Factors that compromise the immune system lower the threshold at which this saturation is reached. A high-fat diet is one such factor.

Promoters are those substances that encourage the growth of cancer cells once they have been formed. A well-known promoter is fat, probably partly because of its immune-suppressing property and partly because its concentrated caloric value encourages growth. Protein is also a likely promoter, since many of the amino acids, once deaminated, are basically bits of fat and are handled as such by the body.

Cancers are usually named according to the organs they affect. The promoters of all types seem to be pretty much the same; the initiators differ depending on the site of entry. Thus, lung cancer is related to smoking and atmospheric pollutants; colon cancer is related to putrefying food particles that are not cleared out by fiber. Breast cancer and prostate cancer seem to be hormone-related, and certain animal products, especially dairy products and beef from slaughtered dairy cows (which is the source of most of the cheap "hamburger" meat in the United States) stimulate excessive hormone release. An excellent book on this latter subject is *Your Life in Your Hands: Understanding, Overcoming and Preventing Breast Cancer* by Dr. Jane A. Plant, who is one of Britain's most distinguished scientists (chief scientist for the British Geological Survey). She states that she overcame a death sentence from breast cancer through diet, principally by elimination of all animal products for eight months. The paperback version of the book is titled *The No-Dairy Breast Cancer Prevention Program*. She documents in detail the rationale for her dietary recommendations, particularly condemning dairy products and the meat from dairy cows. Dr. Plant later wrote another book, *Understanding, Overcoming and Preventing Osteoporosis*, to answer the questions posed to her after she recommended that women eliminate all dairy products. Her conclusion in that book is that dairy products, and especially cheese, *contribute* to bone loss, rather than prevent it, because of their high protein and acidifying effect on the blood. Another book that examines the relationship between animal product consumption and chronic disease risk is *The China Study* by Dr. T. Colin Campbell, professor emeritus in nutrition at Cornell University. This book presents results of a major epidemiological study and also expounds in detail the various stages of cancer progression that casein, the major protein in cow's milk, inhibits the body's immune system from being able to stop. See Addenda 2 and 3 at the end of this book for some of the research evidence presented in these books and other articles linking animal product consumption, especially dairy, to breast, prostate, and ovarian cancer risk.

Another suspect in cancer causation is viruses. There are cancer-causing viruses in farm animals, and these can be spread by contact with them and consumption of their milk and eggs. It has been shown that these are transmissible not only within species but also between different species of animals. This is fully documented in a book by medical doctors Agatha and Calvin Thrash called *The Animal Connection*.

Some factors in foods seem to be protective against certain types of cancers. Fiber's role in helping prevent colon cancer is widely accepted. Cruciferous (cabbage family) vegetables contain a substance called sulforaphane, which seems to enhance the body's production of some cancer-fighting enzymes. Vitamins A (as beta-carotene only), C, E, and the trace mineral selenium—all antioxidants—have been associated with lower cancer risks, especially esophageal, stomach, and lung cancer. These are epidemiological reports from areas where these nutrients are consumed in plentiful amounts from foods, not supplements.

NOTES

[17] Expounded by K.K. Carroll in "Dietary Protein and Heart Disease" in *Nutrition and the M.D.*, June 1985.

[18] "Fats and Cholesterol," Harvard School of Public Health, "The Nutrition Source," accessed January 12, 2015, http://www.hsph.harvard.edu/nutritionsource/what-should-you-eat/fats-and-cholesterol/.

Practice Test: UNIT 15 — Diet-Related Chronic Disease I

Study the **Information Summary** *and then try to complete this test from memory.**

1. Define the following terms:

   Acute deficiency disease

   Chronic disease

   Ischemia

   Myocardial Infarction

   Atherosclerosis

   Arteriosclerosis

   Coronary Heart Disease

   Stroke

   Hypertension

Practice Test: UNIT 15 — Diet-Related Chronic Disease I

2. How does a vegan diet affect blood pressure? What theory has been proposed to explain why?

3. What is congestive heart failure? Is it caused by excess salt intake?

4. Discuss the difference between initiators and promoters of cancer.

5. List some of the factors in foods that are associated with reduced cancer risks.

*Answer Keys *begin on page 134.*

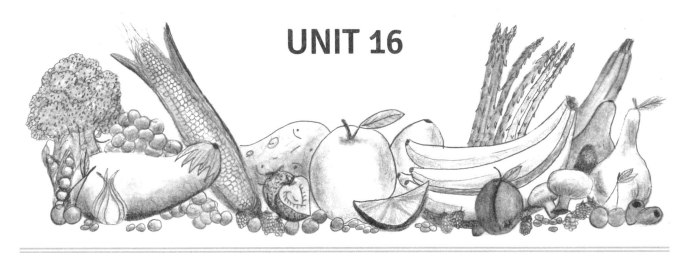

UNIT 16

Diet-Related Chronic Disease II

Information Summary

There are several other chronic disease conditions that have been linked to diet. Some of these that may correlate with animal-derived food consumption are discussed in this unit: diabetes mellitus, kidney failure, osteoporosis, gallstones, and arthritis.

DIABETES

The word diabetes is from the Greek "to siphon," referring to a syndrome in which urination is abnormally frequent and plentiful. In some disorders this urine is of normal constituency (called diabetes insipidus, a condition unrelated to diet), but most often the urine contains significant amounts of glucose, and the condition is then called diabetes mellitus. "Mellitus" is from the Greek word for "sweet," while "insipidus" literally means "tasteless," indications of the bravery of the physicians of long ago who actually sampled their patients' copious specimens. There are now, of course, chemical indicator kits available.

Insulin is a hormone produced by the pancreas. The function of insulin is to alert the cells of the body that the blood glucose level has reached a high level and to encourage those cells to take in some of the glucose and use it as a present or future (stored as fat) energy source. The precipitating event of diabetes mellitus is a lack of insulin or ineffectiveness of insulin to rid the blood of excess glucose. Some of the latter is excreted into the urine (normally calorie-containing molecules aren't excreted) in an attempt to lower the blood glucose level. This glucose spillage into the urine doesn't usually get rid of enough to check the rising blood concentration, but it does provide an excellent indicator for diagnostic purposes.

The reason high blood glucose levels are dangerous is not merely because of the abnormal urination, but rather because of the effect of the high sugar concentration on small capillaries in the body. The proteins on the walls of these capillaries become glycosylated. This means that glucose attaches to them, eventually hardening them much like rock candy that forms on a string dipped into a melted sugar solution. These glycosylated proteins are then unable to expand and contract as blood flow dictates and can easily burst. This compromises the function of the organ system in which they are located. This most frequently seems to occur in the eyes (diabetes is the most common cause of blindness in the United States), the kidneys (25% of all kidney failure is caused by diabetes), and in the heart (diabetes sufferers have more than twice the rate of heart disease as nondiabetics).

Most people with diabetes mellitus (approximately 90%–95%) have what is called noninsulin-dependent diabetes mellitus (NIDDM), sometimes referred to as adult-onset, or type II, diabetes. The other principal form is type I or "juvenile" diabetes, more accurately called insulin-dependent diabetes mellitus (IDDM). The difference obviously is whether the individual needs insulin injections to control his or her disease (IDDM) or can control it with diet alone (NIDDM). In the former case, the situation is one in which the pancreas fails to secrete adequate insulin, while the latter is one in which the insulin is produced but lacks effectiveness.

In NIDDM, the reasons for which insulin loses its effectiveness have not been clearly elucidated. One theory is that fats may block the insulin message from reaching the cells. Another theory is that the cells just ignore the message in their desperate attempt to burn the fats. These suggestions come from studies of populations that switch from the high complex-carbohydrate diet typical of "less developed" countries to the high fat diet typical of modern societies. The rate of NIDDM often goes up dramatically. (The research of Cornell University's T. Colin Campbell in China has shown this to be directly correlated with meat consumption.) Some populations seem much more prone to development of the disease, indicating a genetic factor in predisposition to it. However, it does not become widespread until a rich diet is adopted.

Once an individual has diabetes mellitus, it is carbohydrates (especially refined ones) that will cause the blood sugar to go even higher. Because of this fact, the misconception exists that carbohydrates are the cause of the disease in the first place. Quite the reverse is true: the cause is likely the replacement of carbohydrate calories with fat and protein calories. Another reason for the misconception is that most often refined carbohydrates are eaten laden with added fats: pies, cakes, soft candies, cookies, ice cream, bread with butter, etc. The carbohydrates get implicated because they get left in the blood to cause damage as the body attempts to deal with the fats. The fact that the fiber is also removed from the foods adds to the problem.

Dietary treatment of diabetes mellitus has traditionally focused merely on the carbohydrate content of foods. This was supposed to serve as an indication of the amount of glucose that would eventually end up in the blood. A more recent approach has been to evaluate individual foods according to their actual glycemic ("glucose in blood") effect. Thus, foods are rated according to a glycemic index: the higher the number, the higher the blood glucose peak reached by human subjects eating that food. Interesting results have been obtained, indicating that factors such as cooking time and method, fat content, and of course fiber can greatly affect glycemic response. For instance, two high-carbohydrate foods that have unexpectedly low glycemic index numbers are beans and ice cream, the former because of their high soluble fiber content (good) and the latter because of its high fat content (bad). On the other hand, many were surprised to see that both white bread and whole wheat bread have equal and very high glycemic index numbers. Starch is apparently converted to glucose very quickly, and the fiber in whole wheat flour is so finely ground that it does not slow the process. As far as sweeteners go, fructose ranks much lower than sucrose, and honey (because it has already been digested once by a bee) is much higher than both.

The less common type of diabetes mellitus, Type I, or juvenile diabetes, is characterized by a severe lack of insulin production by the pancreas. The treatment is insulin replacement through daily injections. It has always been considered purely a genetic disorder, unrelated to diet or other lifestyle factors. A study done in the early 1990s in Toronto (ironically the same city in which insulin treatment was developed decades earlier) cites cow's milk as one factor that sets off the destruction of the insulin-making tissue of the pancreas early in life.[19] The study, headed by Dr. Hans-Michael Dosch of the Hospital for Sick Children, shows that when cow's milk is not given to those babies considered genetically predisposed to IDDM for at least their first nine months, the disease is not likely to develop.

Hypoglycemia is a condition in which the blood glucose falls abnormally low on an intermittent but regular basis. This can cause symptoms such as weakness and "inward trembling." Many experts consider this an early warning of diabetes mellitus (which will manifest as hyperglycemia). Hypo means "below" [normal]; hyper means "above" [normal]. It is postulated that hypoglycemia occurs because insulin is released too long after eating, by which time much of the glucose absorbed from the meal has been burned for calories. This is most likely to happen when the foods eaten are quickly absorbed. The best dietary treatment for hypoglycemia is to eat foods that delay the release of glucose into the blood, the most healthful of which are those with adequate intact fiber (all vegan of course). Diabetics (and hypoglycemic persons) formerly were instructed to eat a diet rich in fats and protein and avoid carbohydrates. Since diabetes often leads to heart disease and kidney problems, this is no longer considered appropriate.

KIDNEY FAILURE

Kidney and liver diseases can result from a lifetime of stress on these organs from high-protein diets. One group of kidney diseases, collectively called **nephrotic syndrome**, involves a great loss of body protein into the urine. (The functioning unit of the kidneys is called **nephrons**, of which there are approximately one million in each kidney.) The nephrons normally allow only the smaller molecules of waste material through for excretion. The large molecules of body protein are supposed to get screened back into the blood stream. It was traditionally believed that the best way to treat this was with a high-protein diet (1.5 g/kg body weight) in an attempt to replace lost body proteins. It is now recognized that a lower level of protein (0.6 g/kg body weight, actually less than the normal RDA of 0.8 g/kg) replaces lost body protein just as well and slows the loss. Obviously the lower dietary protein levels give the kidneys a rest and a chance to heal.

The outer portions of the kidneys were probably not intended to have to work all the time. Our ancestors evolved eating a largely vegan diet, with an occasional meat meal when a dead animal was stumbled upon. Even after hunting evolved (probably in times of scarcity) a kill was made once every few weeks, and meat was eaten for a day or two until it rotted. Handling a heavy protein load on a regular basis is a very modern situation, one to which our kidneys have yet to adapt. Thus, the outer layers (cortex) of the kidneys, designed to function on only an intermittent basis, are overworked to the point of **sclerosis**. Eventually even the inner layers are overburdened and wear out as well. Chronic renal failure, a complete shutdown of all kidney function, is the result.[20]

Chronic renal failure has long been treated with what is called a "low-protein diet." This diet actually contains 20 to 40 grams of protein. It is thus not deficient, just adequate without being excessive. Many kidney patients who stick with this diet (almost purely vegan) get and stay better. Those who don't wind up on artificial kidney machines (dialysis) often for the rest of their (shortened) lives.

OSTEOPOROSIS

The loss of calcium from bones results in osteoporosis. High protein and high phosphorus intakes can be contributing factors, as can repeated overdoses of pre-formed vitamins A and/or D.[21] A high-fat diet can also contribute, since fats can form "soaps" with calcium, rendering it unable to be absorbed. Some or all of these situations are likely with an animal-product-centered diet. The epidemic proportions of its incidence are such that osteoporosis now affects one out of three Americans over the age of 65 and many younger people as well. Other factors that can contribute to calcium loss are cigarette smoking, excessive caffeine, alcohol, or refined carbohydrates consumption, lack of exercise, and prolonged use of certain medications such as aluminum-containing antacids, steroids, tetracycline, and exogenous thyroid hormone.

It is often considered a "woman's disease," but it affects males in approximately one in eight cases. Men are less likely to develop it at the same age as women because they usually have a larger bone mass and therefore can afford to lose more of it before the disease causes fragility. Women are much more likely to develop it after menopause because the sex hormone estrogen has a calcium-retentive effect. This is probably so because as long as the woman's body thinks there is a possibility of a pregnancy, it holds on to calcium more dearly as a reserve for building an infant skeleton. Younger women who have their ovaries removed are also more likely to develop osteoporosis, since they lose their estrogen-making capability. These facts lead to the odd but common notion that osteoporosis is caused by an estrogen "deficiency" and that the cure is estrogen replacement. While this may help slow calcium loss temporarily (with possible severe side effects), the real roots of the problem are not addressed.

GALLSTONES

The formation of gallstones (concretions usually composed of calcium/cholesterol that block the flow of bile from the gall bladder into the small intestine) is much more likely in nonvegans than in vegans. Obviously the cholesterol connection may be similar to that involved in the development of atherosclerosis. Another contributing factor may be the effect of a high phosphorus diet. Since the effect of phosphorus is to lower the blood calcium but not necessarily excrete it (as excessive protein does), there is a tendency for some of the calcium to get deposited in soft tissues. This phenomenon is called **calcification**. Stone formation may then result.

Some research (meat industry–sponsored) has shown that meat causes less calcium excretion into the urine than might be predicted based on its protein content. The conclusion is then made that the phosphorus in the meat prevents the loss. In truth it may be just that the phosphorus channels some of the calcium into soft tissue areas, such as the gall bladder, kidneys, or lungs. The net loss of calcium from bone is the same as predicted, and other problems become a risk as well.

ARTHRITIS

Inflammation of the joints is referred to as **arthritis**. It is a symptom, not a disease, but it is so widespread and causes such discomfort that coping with it has become an end in itself. The cause of arthritis is officially listed as "unknown." The most common forms of chronic arthritis are labeled **osteoarthritis, rheumatoid arthritis,** and **gout**.

Osteoarthritis, sometimes called degenerative arthritis, is the most common form. It occurs more frequently in obese people, who suffer severe stress in weight-bearing joints (knees, hips, ankles, spine). It also occurs (actually most commonly) in finger and thumb joints. When obese people lose weight, their arthritis gets better not just in the weight-bearing joints but in the hands as well. This indicates that it is not just the stress of weight that causes the disease but something in the diet as well (possibly fat, since obese people often get that way by overdoing lipids). Non-obese arthritis sufferers often report improvement with dietary change, which usually involves a reduction in fats, especially those from animal products.

Rheumatoid arthritis is more severe than osteoarthritis, is most common in the hands and feet, and is characterized by swelling of the joints. It occurs in the underweight as frequently as the overweight. Since this type of joint pain can be a symptom of a food allergy, dietary change sometimes has a profound effect. Dairy products, the most common human food allergen, are one likely candidate as a contributing causative factor. An "elimination diet" is the best way to detect a food allergy. This is a diet in which all but the most nonallergenic foods (such as rice, pears, carrots) are avoided for two weeks or until symptoms disappear. Then, suspected allergens are eaten (challenged) for a day or two each to see if any bring symptoms back. If no improvement is noted in the two weeks or so on the elimination diet, chances are there is no food allergy involved.

Gout is less common but has been persistently recorded as a disorder for hundreds of years. It has always been related to a "rich" diet, since it is characterized by accumulation of **uric acid** in the blood. Uric acid is a breakdown product of **purines**, which are a part of DNA and RNA (nucleoproteins). The organs and blood of animals are rich in purines; thus liver, meat extracts, and fish that are eaten whole (sardines, anchovies, scallops) are to be avoided by people with this condition. Usually the body clears uric acid out into the urine, but those who lose the ability to do so adequately risk having sodium urate crystals form around the joints, causing a gouty arthritis. Gout is considered a hereditary condition, but those with the propensity toward it will usually not have problems if they avoid a rich diet. The only vegan food rich in purines is yeast (brewer's, baker's, and nutritional). Using these excessively (more than approximately two tablespoons daily) is not recommended for those with a family history of gout. (If one is not sure whether this disorder runs in the family, it is prudent to limit supplemental yeast intake anyway.)

NOTES

[19] HC Gerstein, "Cow's milk exposure and type I diabetes mellitus. A critical overview of the clinical literature," *Diabetes Care* 17, no. 1 (January 1994): 13-9.

[20] Barry M. Brenner, Timothy W. Meyer, and Thomas H. Hostetter, "Dietary Protein Intake and the Progressive Nature of Kidney Disease," *The New England Journal of Medicine* 307, no. 11 (1982): 652.

[21] For some of the original research done in this regard, see "High-Protein Diets and Bone Homeostasis," *Nutrition Reviews* 39, no. 1 (January 1981): 11–13.

Practice Test: UNIT 16 — Diet-Related Chronic Disease II

Study the **Information Summary** *and then try to complete this test from memory.**

1. Distinguish between the two major types of diabetes mellitus.

2. How do you respond to someone who claims that he or she can't be a vegan because "all those carbohydrates will bring out my diabetes"?

3. Why is a food's glycemic index not merely a reflection of its carbohydrate content?

4. What is the connection recently noted between cow's milk and diabetes?

5. Why was it formerly thought that some people with kidney disease needed a lot more protein than recommended for normal people, instead of less, as is now usually given?

Practice Test: UNIT 16 — Diet-Related Chronic Disease II

6. What might explain why vegans are less prone to gallstones than meat-eaters?

7. List four factors (they don't all have to be related to diet) that could contribute to development of osteoporosis.

8. What are the three common types of arthritis?

    i.

    ii.

    iii.

9. Describe an "elimination diet" and what it might be used for detecting.

*Answer Keys *begin on page 134.*

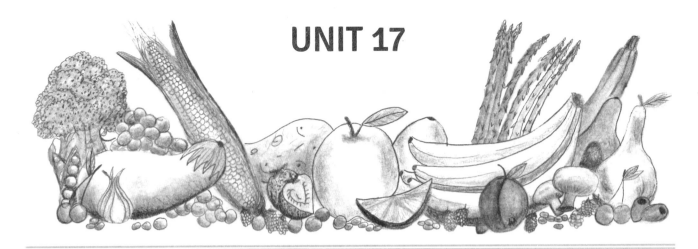

UNIT 17

Life Cycle & Veganism

Information Summary

The stages in the human life cycle are pregnancy, lactation, infancy, childhood, adulthood, and old age. Most of what has been discussed in this book so far has addressed the adulthood stage. Many health professionals believe that the other stages are the ones that present the most nutritional risk, and so have reservations about endorsing alternative diets, including veganism, during those stages. Sometimes vegans themselves hesitate to stay with their diet during pregnancy and sometimes balk at encouraging their children to follow it, all out of fear of inadequate nutriture. Although entire college-level nutrition courses are devoted to life cycle needs, only a basic understanding of nutrition, combined with knowledge of the content of vegan foods, ought to be enough to allay that fear. It also helps to know some healthy second- and third-generation vegans, of which there are many. (For some shining examples, see the photographs in *Pregnancy, Children and the Vegan Diet* by Michael Klaper, MD.)

PREGNANCY

The nutritional status of a woman before she even conceives a child is actually more important to having a healthy baby than is her diet during pregnancy. However, diet during pregnancy is important, both for the health of the infant and that of the mother. As recently as the early 1960s, many health professionals believed that encouraging a smaller-sized newborn through restriction of maternal diet was a proper way to ensure an easier delivery. This stemmed from the idea that the fetus was basically a parasite that would take what it needed from the mother's stores. Statistics have since borne out that this can lead to premature births and possibly birth defects, so it is no longer done. We now know the growing fetus is not a parasite, especially in the first four months or so of pregnancy. Nature does not let the mother's nutritional status get dangerously deficient. Thus, more attention is now paid to providing the materials for building a healthy baby.

While there is an increased need for many nutrients, very few nutrient needs are actually doubled in pregnancy. Calorie needs, for instance, are only about 15% higher for a woman who starts out at a normal weight. Thus, the idea of "eating for two" can lead to excess weight gain. Many obese adult women trace their weight gain back to their pregnancies. The 15% increase in calories is designed to result in the recommended weight gain of 22 to 28 pounds over the nine-month term. Women who start out underweight when they get pregnant may be encouraged to gain slightly more than this and so may eat a few more kcals. Overweight women may be encouraged to gain less weight, so calorie intake would be lower, possibly even at the same level as pre-pregnancy. It is not advisable, though, for an overweight woman to try to lose weight while pregnant.

There are two significant things that happen during pregnancy that affect the need for essential nutrients. First, the woman's body shifts to a more efficient absorption level of those nutrients not usually absorbed at 100%. This is especially relevant to calcium and iron, both of which are absorbed at approximately double the nonpregnant rate. The second thing is that menstruation stops, so the usual monthly loss of blood containing significant amounts of iron, among other nutrients, is kept in the body.

In spite of these factors, however, the recommendation is usually made for supplementation with iron. This is an outgrowth of the prevalence of anemia in pregnant women in North America. A likely explanation for the occurrence of this anemia is that pregnant women are told to drink lots of cow's milk, usually at least four glasses a day. This low-iron food also has the effect of causing iron loss to those who are even slightly allergic to or intolerant of it (through gastrointestinal bleeding). The irony is that milk is pushed for the mistaken idea that extra calcium is needed. It isn't, since it gets absorbed more effectively. In trying to prevent one deficiency, another may be created. Vitamin D needs are no higher in pregnancy (the extra calcium absorption apparently is not mediated by vitamin D), so this cannot be used as an excuse for encouraging milk, either.

Protein needs are slightly higher: the RDA for pregnant women is 60 g (compared to 44 g for nonpregnant women). This is easily achieved on a vegan diet. The nutrient of usual concern for vegans—vitamin B-12— is needed at a level only 10% higher than in the nonpregnant state. Cobalamin, presumably because of its mineral nature (remember it contains the trace element cobalt), is not usually absorbed very well; absorption increases during pregnancy.

The only nutrient for which the RDA is actually more than doubled from the nonpregnant state is folacin. This B-vitamin is needed for building red blood cells, many of which are needed to stock the infant's blood supply. Other blood-building nutrients—iron, copper, cobalamin (B-12)—can be stored in the body and can be absorbed at greater levels during pregnancy.

Folacin is not stored to any great extent and is normally absorbed at a near 100% rate. Thus, intake must be higher and regular. It has recently been noted that pregnant women with low intakes of folacin are more at risk of having babies with a common birth defect called **spina bifida**. This is a condition in which the spinal column fails to form properly. For this reason some health practitioners, especially in Canada, recommend higher-than-RDA doses of folacin for pregnant women.

LACTATION

Lactation, the flow of breast milk for infant feeding, begins immediately after delivery. The naturalness of this process is exemplified by the fact that women who choose not to breastfeed must be given an injection of a drug that inhibits the milk flow. The first flow from the breast after delivery is a slightly more watery version of breast milk called colostrum, which is loaded with antibodies that will help the newborn resist the contagious diseases to which the mother has been exposed. It also contains bifidus factors, substances that promote the growth of "friendly" bacteria in the infant's otherwise sterile intestine. For these reasons women are often encouraged to breastfeed for at least a day or two after giving birth, although it seems that at least six months of breastfeeding is required before full immunity against disease and allergy is obtained.

For those women who do choose to breastfeed, the sucking of the infant is usually all that is needed to keep a woman's body producing milk for up to six years. Most women in modern societies (La Leche League excepted) do stop after a year or two. At that time the flow begins to decline slightly and soon dries up completely if nursing is discontinued.

The nutrient needs of the lactating woman are generally slightly greater than during pregnancy. The RDAs for protein, vitamins A and E, thiamin, riboflavin, niacin, cobalamin, Mg, I, Zn, and Se are increased on the order of 10%–20%. The RDAs for calcium and vitamins D and K are the same as during pregnancy (actually the same as in the pre-pregnant state as well). The RDAs for folacin, pyridoxine, and iron are lower than during pregnancy. Even for lactating women, the RDAs do not necessarily reflect true needs, especially in regard to those who do not consume a typical Western high-protein diet. The need for calcium by lactating women consuming a less excessive level of protein was explored in a 1995 study published in the *American Journal of Clinical Nutrition*.[22] The authors experimented on a group of breastfeeding women in the African nation of Gambia. These women were receiving only about 300 mg of calcium (compared to the American RDA of 1,200 mg) daily from their diet, which was principally vegan. These women were then given a supplement containing an additional 714 mg. It was found that no additional calcium was detected in the mothers' milk or their bones, meaning that they were probably already getting enough.

VEGAN POINT OF INFORMATION

In one of the landmark studies of vegans, Dr. T.A.B. Sanders of the University of London followed the pregnancies of 50 vegan mothers. Not only did they all give birth to normal, healthy babies, but all those who chose to do so went on to successfully breastfeed their infants.[23] The nature of lactation is such that serious deficiencies in the maternal diet will result in inadequate milk flow, thereby requiring bottle supplementation. Mother Nature generally won't allow an "incomplete" milk to be produced.

One exception some may point to is the published case of an infant in poor health found to be nursed by a vegan mother. The mother's blood level of vitamin B-12 was low, that of her breast milk was low, and that of the infant's blood was low (although his symptoms were not those of classic B-12 deficiency). Nevertheless, on supplementation with B-12, his condition improved greatly, so the conclusion was that this was the problem. The mother was experiencing no ill health in spite of her low blood B-12. The fact that was not stressed was that this infant was 10 months old and was being fed no other foods. The potential for obtaining B-12 from microorganisms on or in food was thus denied, as breast milk itself is sterile. The bifidus factor mentioned above encourages bacterial growth; it is not bacteria itself. The B-12 must be supplied through the environment, usually in foods or other beverages.

It is indeed frustrating how case studies such as this one, flawed as it may be, are used to condemn veganism at certain stages of life. Yet when cases of healthy vegans are cited, these are often dismissed as merely "anecdotal" and therefore not scientific.

INFANCY

The ideal food for human infants is human breast milk. Looking at its constituents, especially compared to cow's milk, provides a good introduction to infant nutrition. The (now mostly lost) art of making formula created infant nutrition experts of those who had to feed the non-breastfed baby. The widespread current use of prepared formulas has virtually eliminated this acquisition of knowledge.

MAKING INFANT FORMULA

In order to make a formula—that is, to substitute cow's milk for human milk—several things must be done or else the infant will not thrive. Firstly, since any protein other than that of human milk is difficult for the infant to digest, the cow's milk must be *heated*. This denatures, or uncoils, the protein strands, making it more easily broken apart by the infant's enzymes. This is necessary for cow's milk as sold in cartons or bottles. Commercial formulas already have the milk protein denatured, as does evaporated (canned) milk. Denaturing does not change the protein content or the amino acid sequence; it merely affects the secondary structure (configuration) of the protein. If the infant is truly allergic to milk protein, denaturing won't help much; a different milk, usually soy, is then used. In many hospitals now, newborns not breastfed are routinely started on soy-based formula to reduce the possibility of having to change.

The second thing that has to be done to cow's milk in creating a formula is to *dilute* it. Compared to human milk, cow's milk has the same number of calories per unit of weight or volume (about 20 kcal per g or cc), but cow's milk has approximately twice as much protein and major mineral content. This is referred to as the renal solute load, or the amount of material with which the kidneys will have to deal. In order to make this load one with which the human infant can deal, a dilution of approximately 2:1 with sterile water is required. It is indeed ironic that the two "growth" nutrients for which milk is usually pushed—calcium and protein—are present in such excessive amounts that they could kill the human infant if left undiluted.

The third thing that needs to be done to create a formula is to *restore calories* to it. In spite of its high protein level, cow's milk has the same caloric density as human milk, approximately 20 kcal/fluid ounce. The difference is that human milk has much more carbohydrate (actually, yes, lactose) than cow's milk. Thus, after dilution, the caloric density is halved, and the human infant would be physically incapable of swallowing enough volume of formula to meet its energy needs. And so, a source of easily digestible carbohydrate, usually corn syrup (mostly glucose) is added. It is again ironic that the same lactose that most adults have trouble digesting is not only present but very abundant in their mothers' milk. Maybe Mother Nature wanted to make sure adults didn't steal stuff meant for the babies in times of shortage.

In summary, then, preparing infant formula necessitates heating cow's milk to denature the protein (and thus make it less allergenic) and then diluting it with water and adding an additional carbohydrate source (like corn syrup). The result is a formula that resembles human milk in terms of these gross parameters, but many other differences still exist. Some of these are somewhat correctable, such as adding more of certain vitamins and trace minerals. Others are not correctable, such as its lack of immunity-granting antibodies and lower absorbability of nutrients.

ENERGY REQUIREMENTS OF INFANTS

The recommended energy intake for infants from zero to six months is approximately 650 kcal/day. Dividing this by 20 kcal/oz yields a recommended consumption of approximately 32 oz (1 qt) of milk or formula, just about what the average lactating woman produces. Mothers of twins produce approximately twice this much. Nature knows. The recommended energy intake for infants from six months to a year is approximately 850 kcal/day, more than the lactating woman can produce (for one infant).

STARTING SOLID FOODS

Once the infant is four or five months old it is considered appropriate to start "solid" foods. These are actually semisolid, at most, because these usually toothless babies cannot chew much. That these foods are liquid is important, not only because of the lack of teeth but also because infants cannot concentrate their wastes well and are obliged to excrete much more water than adults. Feeding dry foods, or even foods with 50% or 60% water content (such as meats and eggs), can cause dehydration. The usual recommended order of introduction of food categories is: cereals, vegetables, fruits, legumes, and then nuts.

The first foods recommended to be introduced are cooked cereals, which are about 85% water when prepared. Rice, the least allergenic, is recommended first. New foods are generally introduced one at a time, waiting at least a day or two in between to note any intolerance. Vegetables are usually recommended next because most of them are less likely to be allergenic than many fruits. Also, some health professionals believe it is better to delay the introduction of the sweeter fruits until the more bland vegetables are accepted. Others say, however, that the natural sweetness of breast milk (and, as a result of carbohydrate addition, formula) indicates that a preference for sweets is probably innate, making it a moot point. The allergy issue, though, may be relevant. The later a potentially allergic food of any category is introduced, the less likely it will cause a problem.

Legumes and their products (tofu, etc.) are introduced next, at no earlier than six months of age, though eight months may be more ideal. Nuts are not recommended until teeth are well in place to avoid choking. Nut butters and milks may be introduced earlier, however. Meats are not recommended until at least nine months of age. (In this guide, obviously, they are not recommended at all.) Eggs and cow's milk (the most allergenic foods) are not recommended until twelve months.

VEGAN POINT OF INFORMATION

A British study (noted in Jean Carper's *Nutrition* syndicated newspaper column on September 23, 1992) found that infants who were not given milk, eggs, fish, or nuts for their first year of life were almost three times less likely to develop allergic conditions such as eczema and asthma. The group studied included both bottle-fed and breast-fed babies. Lactating mothers were instructed to avoid those foods; the same effects were noted.

CHILDHOOD

After one year of life an infant technically becomes a "child." The diet at this stage begins to resemble an adult diet but with special attention given to nutrients needed for growth in stature. One such nutrient that gets all too much attention is calcium. Growing children absorb it at a much greater rate than adults, so forcing large amounts on them (usually in the form of milk) is unnecessary. The RDA for calcium for children is 800 mg from age one to ten and then 1200 mg from age eleven through the teen years. As with adults, these high numbers reflect an attempt to replace calcium that is lost on an inordinate high-protein diet. The child's RDA for vitamin D is double of that recommended for adults. This is best and most easily gotten from sun exposure. Even in cold climates, it has been found that liberal sun exposure during the summer can result in enough vitamin D storage to last through the winter. For those children who do not get sun exposure, though, supplements may be necessary. They do not, again, have to be given at the same time that calcium-rich foods are ingested.

In another study undertaken by Dr. Sanders (along with R. Purves), 25 vegan children under the age of five were measured.[24] Only two children (a brother and sister of short parents) were below normal height for their age. This was in spite of the fact that all of them had calcium intakes that were below recommended levels. It is interesting to examine the protein (the other nutrient often associated with "growth") RDA for infants and children. Remember, for adults it is 0.8 g/kg of body weight. For infants, it starts at a whopping 2.2 g/kg of body weight (easily met with breast milk) from birth to six months. From six months to a year the RDA drops to 1.5 g/kg, providing the opportunity to start feeding lower protein foods like cereals and fruits. In childhood, it drops to 1.2 g/kg from age one to six years, then to 1.0 g/kg from age seven to fourteen years. From age fifteen to eighteen years it goes down to 0.9 g/kg, and after age nineteen, the adult level of 0.8 g/kg is in effect. From this standpoint it is clearer also why fiber's hindrance of protein absorption can be a problem for smaller children. They need more relative to their size, so they need to absorb all the nutrients they eat. The fact that as early as age seven the protein RDA is already only slightly higher than in adulthood (1.0 vs. 0.8 g/kg) indicates how overrated the need for protein-rich foods is. A hearty bowl of cooked cereal three times a day can just about provide the 22 grams of protein recommended for a typical 22 kg (48 lb) seven-year-old. Add a few vegetables and it is well over the RDA.

Remember too, though, that if calories are in short supply, protein will not be used for growth. Recommended calorie intakes for children are shown in Table 17.1. The splits for ages older than eleven in Table 17.1 reflect differences in growth patterns for girls and boys. The lower levels are those recommended for girls. Remember that these are all averages based on typical size and activity. Appetite is the best guide for proper consumption levels provided appropriate foods are made available and an environment free of inordinate stress is present.

Table 17.1 — Recommended Calorie Intakes for Children (United States)	
1–3 years	1,300 kcal/day
4–6 years	1,800 kcal/day
7–10 years	2,000 kcal/day
11–14 years	2,200–2,500 kcal/day
15–18 years	2,200–3,000 kcal/day

ADULTHOOD & OLD AGE

Adulthood is marked by the stoppage of growth in stature, usually occurring at about age 19. This obviously means that nutrition heretofore needed for that growth will be superfluous. An unhealthy weight can occur if calories are not reduced, unless, of course, activity is increased. Given our social patterns, it is likely that activity decreases rather than increases, as the individual starts a usually sedentary job in place of the active life of the schoolyard. Compounding this, on average, it seems that the energy expended for basal metabolism declines by about 5% every decade after age 30, owing largely to reduction of muscle mass.

Old age is considered to be the period after age 65. Nutrient needs during this time are influenced less by biological factors and more by physical factors. Two of these are the loss of teeth for biting and chewing fresh fruits and vegetables and the loss of mobile strength for carrying these heavy foods home from the store. Often, health professionals will recommend that the elderly consume more concentrated sources of nutrients, such as liver and other organ meats, for these reasons. The problems can be more optimally overcome by using a blender or food processor to lessen the need for chewing and also by advising the purchase of smaller quantities of produce at a time. Most markets will gladly divide up prepackaged containers. Encouragement of window box gardening and sprouting is also recommended.

One nutrient sometimes of concern for the elderly is vitamin D. If liver function declines, the ability of the body to manufacture this hormone from sunlight may be compromised. Also, many people begin to avoid the sun completely for fear of wrinkles and/or skin cancer. The result of this deficiency is osteomalacia, not osteoporosis. For those at risk, it has been found that a once-yearly injection of vitamin D (remember, it gets stored) will prevent problems. Supplements are also available but would have to be taken more frequently. Milk drinking is unnecessary, something many lactose-intolerant individuals are delighted to hear.

NOTES

[22] A. Prentice et al., "Calcium requirements of lactating Gambian mothers: effects of a calcium supplement on breast-milk calcium concentration, maternal bone mineral content, and urinary calcium excretion," *American Journal of Clinical Nutrition* 62, no. 1 (July 1995): 58-67.

[23] Mabel Cluer et al., *Vegan Mothers and Children* (Leatherhead, England: Vegan Society Limited, 1981) 28.

[24] See endnote 9.

Practice Test: UNIT 17 — Life Cycle & Veganism

Study the **Information Summary** *and then try to complete this test from memory.**

1. Discuss the concept of why or why not pregnancy should be considered a time to "eat for two."

2. What is the only nutrient for which a good case can be made for more than doubling intake during pregnancy?

3. List three advantages of breast-feeding over formula feeding.

    i.

    ii.

    iii.

4. Number the following foods in order of recommended introduction to infants:

    _____ beans

    _____ fruits

    _____ vegetables

    _____ nuts

    _____ cereals

5. How would you respond to someone who "heard that vegetarian children suffer from stunted growth"?

Practice Test: UNIT 17 — Life Cycle & Veganism

6. How, in general (specific numbers not required), does the RDA for protein change from infancy through childhood into adulthood?

7. What factors contribute to the common occurrence of adulthood being a time of becoming overweight?

8. List two physical factors that often lead to the elderly consuming less fresh fruits and vegetables and ways in which these can be overcome (feel free to be creative).

9. Discuss options for providing vitamin D other than through drinking fortified cow's milk.

*Answer Keys *begin on page 134.*

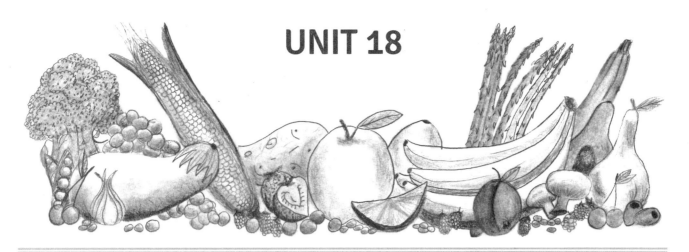

UNIT 18

Summary of Risks & Benefits of Vegan Diets

Information Summary

SUMMARY OF RISKS OF VEGAN DIETS

The nutritional risks usually associated with vegan diets are all associated with being undernourished:

1. Underweight: Because of the higher fiber content of most vegan diets, there is a tendency to eat fewer calories if the same volume of food is eaten. This can easily be overcome (unless one wants to lose weight) by just eating a greater volume of food at each meal and/or by eating more frequent meals.

2. Protein deficiency: Call your local hospital and ask when was the last time they admitted a vegan for treatment of protein deficiency. Compare that to how many people they are treating for kidney failure and for fractures caused by osteoporosis. Perhaps the only times vegans should worry about protein are:
   a. If they are eating an all-fruit diet
   b. If they feed very small children too much fiber, such that protein (and other nutrients) don't get absorbed adequately

3. Iron-deficiency anemia: As mentioned in the unit on Trace Minerals, vegetarians often replace high-iron meats with low-iron dairy products, sometimes resulting in iron-deficiency anemia. Obviously this can be overcome by reducing dairy consumption to a minimum or eliminating it altogether. (A very strong point for veganism.) Iron supplements are also an option, though guesswork (how much is enough and how much is too much) and risk of side effects (such as constipation) are complicating factors.

4. Vitamin B-12 deficiency: This nutrient continues to haunt the vegan diet, yet many more nonvegans than vegans suffer from low blood levels. The prudent thing to do is to assure an occasional supply through fortified foods or supplements, though many vegans continue to live long, healthy, energetic lives without doing so.

SUMMARY OF HEALTH BENEFITS OF A VEGAN DIET

In this book, you have learned about the following health-related advantages of whole plant foods over animal-derived foods.

1. Fiber, a very important but overlooked nutrient, is only found in plant foods.

2. Carbohydrates, the human body's preferred fuel source, are only abundant in plant foods.

3. Plant foods are virtually *free* of artery-clogging cholesterol and, for the most part, are *not rich* in saturated fatty acids: these are the main reasons vegans have lower risk of coronary heart disease, our number one killer disease.

4. Being lower in the food chain, whole plant foods are less contaminated with environmental pollutants, perhaps one of the reasons that vegans have lower risk of certain cancers, our number two killer disease.

5. Vegan foods (other than some heavily refined ones) are not excessive in protein. Excess protein is linked to kidney disease.

6. Animal protein generally has significant amounts of growth hormones—some added, some naturally occurring—that are linked to higher cancer risk.

7. Any one of these issues is enough for health-minded individuals to think about becoming vegan. Collectively they are a powerful argument for anyone even slightly concerned about their own, or their family's, health.

Practice Test: UNIT 18 — Summary of Risks & Benefits of Vegan Diets

Study the **Information Summary** *and then try to complete this test from memory.** *

Summarize the risks and methods for minimizing risks in regard to the following nutrients for vegans.

1. Calories:

2. Protein:

3. Iron:

4. Vitamin B-12 (Cobalamin):

5. Go back to your Practice Test for Unit 3 and look at the last part where you analyzed the energy nutrient composition of a "meal" consisting of the three foods you had chosen.

    Combined percent of calories (round to nearest 1%) as:

    Cholesterol _____%   Fat _____%   Protein _____%

    What would you *now* say about the appropriateness of this balance?

    If not ideal, which food (you may choose one not already on your list) might you add more of to balance it better?

    How much would you add?

*Answer Keys *begin on page 134.*

ANSWER KEYS

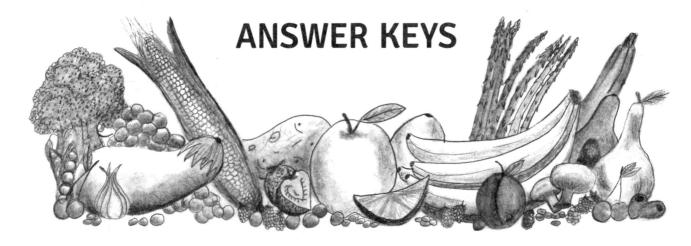

Practice Test: UNIT 1 — Protein: Quality

ANSWER KEY

1. c

2. b

3. b

4. The EAA in shortest supply relative to human need.

5. The amount of a protein that theoretically would be used by the body, derived by the percentage, relative to need, of its limiting EAA.

6. Other factors such as the digestibility of the food are integral to its quality.

7. Outdated studies on rats were used to determine their "completeness." We now know that human beings need much less protein and can get all of the essential amino acids from any one plant protein, as long as enough food is eaten to meet caloric needs.

8. d

Practice Test: UNIT 2 — Protein: Quantity

ANSWER KEY

1. The removal of the amino group from amino acids such that the remaining portions can be used as a source of energy (calories). It occurs in the liver.

2. a. The liver is flooded with the excess amino acids and must work hard to deaminate them all. The ammonia that is broken off forces the liver to engorge itself with fluid (hypertrophy) to dilute it. The liver converts the ammonia into urea and sends it to the kidneys, which also undergo hypertrophy to dilute this harsh substance.

2. b. In order to excrete the urea, the kidneys must take calcium from the blood. To keep the blood calcium constant, bone material is dissolved into it, eventually leading to osteoporosis.

3. b

4. a

5. a

6. When carbohydrates are in short supply, the body will deaminate protein in order to supply glucose to the brain. When adequate CHO is present, protein is preserved and thus allowed to be used for tissue-building functions.

7. Lactose intolerance is an inability to break down the sugar in milk. It results in gastrointestinal upset, such as cramping, diarrhea, or gas production. Milk allergy occurs when the protein in milk enters the bloodstream intact and triggers an allergic reaction. This can manifest itself in any of several body systems: skin rashes, respiratory problems, headache, irritability, etc.

8. b

Practice Test: UNIT 3 — Carbohydrates

ANSWER KEY

Part I

1. e

2. a; m

3. l

4. k

5. j

6. b

7. f

8. g

9. h

10. i

11. d

12. c

13. Carbohydrates' sole function is to serve as a source of energy (calories). Thus, they are misconstrued as "empty calories."

Part II *(Please pardon the algebra...it won't happen again.)*

	Type of Food	Serving Size	Grams of CHO	Grams of Protein	Grams of Fat
Food 1	(varies)	(varies)	a	b	c
Food 2	(varies)	(varies)	d	e	f
Food 3	(varies)	(varies)	g	h	i

Number of calories from:	CHO	Protein	Fat	Total Calories Per Serving
Food 1	4a	4b	9c	(4a + 4b + 9c) = J
Food 2	4d	4e	9f	(4d + 4e + 9f) = K
Food 3	4g	4h	9i	(4g + 4h + 9i) = L
Totals	(4a + 4d + 4g)	(4b + 4e + 4h)	(9c + 9f + 9i)	(J + K + L) = M
(list above)	Total CHO	Total Protein	Total Fat	Total of All Three

Meal 1—Total kcal: (J + K + L) = M

To find energy nutrient percentages of this meal it is necessary to total the grams of each nutrient (don't just total the percentages), thus:

Total CHO grams = a + d + g; let this be represented by n; then total CHO kcalories is 4n, so meal percentage of CHO calories is 100(4n/M) = %CHO

Total protein grams = b + e + h; call this p; total protein kcal is 4p; meal %PROT. = 100(4p/M)

Total fat grams = c + f + I; call this q; total fat kcal is 9q; meal %FAT = 100(9q/M)

Practice Test: UNIT 4 — Fiber

ANSWER KEY

1. To spread the fiber intake throughout the day and to get the fiber from a variety of plant foods. The former to allow the functions of fiber, such as regulating digestive passage, blood sugar, and cholesterol levels, to occur continually; and the latter to assure all types of fiber are consumed, some of which perform one or more functions better than others.

2. *Simple CHO*—Monosaccharides and disaccharides: sugars.

   Complex CHO—Polysaccharides: starch, glycogen, and most fiber in plants.

   Refined CHO—Foods that contain sugars and/or starch but have had most or all of their fiber removed. These may be totally purified carbohydrates, such as white sugar or cornstarch, or have many other nutrients still remaining, such as white rice or fruit juice.

   Unrefined CHO—Whole plant foods with their fiber content intact.

Practice Test: UNIT 5 — Lipids

ANSWER KEY

1. c

2. Linoleic

3. There is adequate EFA in whole plant foods, including vegetables; there is no need to consume fats in isolated form.

4. i. Carrying fat-soluble vitamins: done quite well by whole plant foods, such as vitamin A in carrots.
   ii. Providing a feeling of satiety: can be done with fiber, without also providing a concentrated calorie source.

5. a

6. b

7. c

8. d

9. d

10. c

11. b

12. a

13. It is a chemical process wherein unsaturated fats have hydrogen atoms forced onto their places of unsaturation (double bonds) rendering them saturated; this is done to create a more solid fat with a longer shelf life.

14.

Food	# Calories	Grams of Fat	% Calories From Fat
Potato chips	150	10	$90 \div 150 = 60\%$
Pretzels	100	1	$9 \div 100 = 9\%$

[Note: These are real numbers. Obviously not all snack foods are "created" equal.]

15. i. Excessive intake of saturated triglycerides
    ii. Excessive intake of dietary cholesterol
    iii. Low intake of soluble fiber

16. Blood cholesterol

17. High-density lipoproteins and low-density lipoproteins; the former contain relatively less lipid so are less likely to drop off artery-clogging cholesterol to cause blockage (atherosclerosis).

18. Unsaturated fatty acids that have their first double bond at the third and sixth positions from the methyl end. The ones important nutritionally are the essential fatty acids alpha-linolenic acid and linoleic acid.

Practice Test: UNIT 6 — Digestion & Absorption

ANSWER KEY

1. b

2. e

3. d

4. f

5. l

6. a

7. g

8. j

9. i

10. k

11. c

12. h

13. e

14. a

15. b

16. c

17. d

18. It is the burning sensation that occurs in the lower esophagus when stomach acid backs up through the cardiac sphincter. The esophagus does not have a thick mucus lining to protect it like the stomach does. It is caused by overeating, especially fatty foods, made worse by lying down.

19. b

20. a

21. c

22. d

23. f

24. Stress hormones that cause heavy stomach acid secretion (to help digestion while an animal concentrates its energy on fighting and/or running away) may still be in meat when eaten, causing a similar secretion response. High levels of stomach acid can ulcerate the duodenum when released through the pylorus.

Practice Test: UNIT 7 — Weight Control

ANSWER KEY

1. c

2. lower

3. *R = Raise L = Lower*:

    __R__ Childhood (Growth)

    __R__ Pregnancy

    __L__ Starvation

    __L__ Strict dieting

    __L__ Fasting

    __R__ Fever

    __R__ Lactation

4. c

5. b

6. d

7. c

8. b; $365 \div 20 = 18.25$ pounds will be gained.

9. **BME** = 0.9 (BMR for women) × 50 kg × 24 hrs. = 1,080 kcal

    VAE = 80% × 1,080 (BME) = 864 kcal

    DIT = 10% of 2,000 kcal eaten = 200 kcal

    Total Calorie Expenditure = 1,080 + 864 + 200 = 2,144 kcal

    Rate of Gain or Loss of Fat =
    Calorie deficit of 2,144 - 2,000 = 144 kcal daily
    3,500 kcal in pound of body fat ÷ 144 = 24.3 days to lose one such pound
    Thus, she will lose one pound about every three and a half weeks.

Practice Test: UNIT 8 — Fat-Soluble Vitamins

ANSWER KEY

1. Vitamins A, D, E and K

2. The vitamin A in plants is in the form of beta-carotene, which is not harmful in excess. Pre-formed vitamin A, found in animal products and many supplements, can be toxic in excess.

3. Because both function in the breakdown stage of bone growth, excesses of either can cause loss of bone density, or osteoporosis.

4. Vitamin E

5. Vitamin K

6. b

7. d

8. a

9. c

10. Children, because they are growing.

Practice Test: UNIT 9 — Water-Soluble Vitamins

ANSWER KEY

1. Cobalamin (B-12)

2. e

3. d

4. b

5. c

6. a

7. Because it can mask a cobalamin deficiency. One of the functions of cobalamin is to help activate folacin in its red blood cell formation function. A flood of folacin can overcome this lack of activation, curing the anemia, but the other consequences of cobalamin deficiency, including nerve degeneration, continue without immediate overt symptoms.

8. Only about 10 mg a day are needed to prevent scurvy. The US RDA is 55–60 mg. It has been found that tissue saturation occurs at about 100 mg a day, meaning the body just can't hold any more, although this occurs at more like 150 mg for smokers. Symptoms of overdose (diarrhea) don't occur until one reaches a level of about 3,000 mg a day. Dr. Pauling's recommendations, especially to prevent cancer, are in the range of 10,000 to 12,000 mg a day. He says that patients with cancer do not get diarrhea even at these levels. However, there are reports of pregnant women who habitually take above 2,000 mg a day giving birth to infants who develop scurvy unless given similarly high doses and slowly weaned off them.

9. In a less-than-sterile environment, B-12 is pervasive. For those who are concerned, fortified foods or supplements are available and inexpensive. The fact that many foods are enriched and/or fortified in the typical Western diet (such as vitamin D added to milk) indicates that these diets are not considered "perfect" by nutrition experts, either. The benefits of a vegan diet (low fat, moderate protein, high fiber, low levels of environmental contamination) far outweigh the "hassle" of having to deal with this micronutrient cobalamin.

10. It should have some form of at least these three: thiamin (usually as thiamin mononitrate), riboflavin, and niacin (usually as niacinamide).

11. Some of the vitamins (particularly B vitamins) are needed to metabolize the energy nutrients (CHO, protein, fat) as they function as co-enzymes in metabolic pathways. Also, in helping cure anemia there is an improvement in symptoms such as listlessness and fatigue.

Practice Test: UNIT 10 — Major Minerals I

ANSWER KEY

1. Minerals are inorganic elements; they cannot be broken down or created in any animal or plant body. They must ultimately come from the earth, from which they are taken up into plants. In food preparation, minerals cannot be destroyed, but they can be removed (by milling off outer layers, for instance) or soaked out. If soaked out, the water they are soaked in will always contain what is missing.

2. Major minerals are needed, by human adults, in amounts greater than 100 milligrams daily. Trace minerals are needed in much lesser amounts (50 mg or less per day).

3. Because it is assumed that Americans consume a large amount of protein and thus need more calcium to help make up for its incurred loss.

4. a

5. Osteoporosis is loss of bone density, resulting in brittleness, and is caused by excess calcium loss. This can be a result of excess intake of protein, vitamins A or D, or phosphorus, or from other factors such as lack of exercise. A deficiency of calcium results in the same disorders as vitamin D deficiency: rickets in children and osteomalacia in adults. These disorders are characterized by a softening of bone.

6. Substances in the fiber of certain foods, they have the potential to attach themselves to minerals (especially calcium, iron, and zinc) and render them unable to be absorbed by the body. The most notorious of these binders are phytic acid (found in most whole grains) and oxalic acid (particularly present in spinach and rhubarb). While the effects of these are potentially significant, these effects seem to show up more under laboratory conditions than they do in the real world.

7. Calcium is plentiful in green vegetables and adequate in many other plant-derived foods. It is needed in much lower amounts if one does not eat a high-protein diet (one containing lots of milk, for instance). Adequate vitamin D can easily be manufactured with brief sun exposure. The vitamin D necessary to absorb the calcium moving down the intestine must already have been in the bloodstream for a while; what is present with that calcium (in milk, for instance) is useless at that stage.

8. Meat is high in protein and phosphorus, two factors that in excess lead to calcium loss from bone. In addition, meat has very little calcium to help replace what is lost.

9. Magnesium

10. Sulfur is contained in the essential amino acid methionine (as well as in two nonessential amino acids); it is technically impossible to incur a sulfur deficiency without also having a protein deficiency.

Practice Test: UNIT 11 — Major Minerals II & Water

ANSWER KEY

1. Water travels from the less concentrated area to the more concentrated one in an effort to make both equal.

2. Inside + = Potassium   Inside - = Phosphate
   Outside + = Sodium   Outside - = Chloride

3. Water, sodium, and chloride are essential nutrients.

4. 40%; 60%

5. Sodium bicarbonate; hydrochloric acid

6. d

7. The body is fooled into thinking there is a deficiency of sodium. The kidneys react by withholding sodium and excreting water in order to raise the relative concentration of sodium. This excreted water always has a certain concentration of ions in it, but the kidneys make sure that the cations to be lost are K+, not Na+. So along with the water, potassium is lost and must be replenished.

8. Mushrooms, tomatoes, potatoes, green beans, and strawberries are all richer in potassium than bananas.

9. c

10. c

11. d

12. d

13. c

14. The fact that we normally excrete so much water each day makes it much more appropriate that we eat foods with a higher water content than our bodies have. Just eating meat (55% water, same as us) leaves no extra fluid for excretion, thereby obliging us to drink more water. This may be no pure rationale for veganism, but since it is getting harder and harder to find pure, unpolluted water, any diet that obliges us to find more of it is a minus in that regard.

15. K: Na ratio is 0.2; ideal is more like 4.0, so this food is very unbalanced in this regard.

Pratice Test: UNIT 12 — Trace Minerals

ANSWER KEY

1. They often consume too much dairy and/or eggs, none of which are good sources of iron. To replace meat iron, plant products must be consumed, especially those with high ascorbic acid contents.

2. Iron in plant foods can be absorbed at nearly the same level as meat iron if sufficient vitamin C is still present in the foods.

3. Enlarged thyroid gland from iodine deficiency (similar condition also caused by iodine excess)

4. i. Fortified salt (especially heavy use thereof in fast foods)
   ii. Dairy products that may have traces of iodine medications that are frequently used on cow udders to treat mastitis
   iii. Iodate dough conditioners in commercially baked goods

5. By using yeast-raised products, as yeast inactivates the phytates

6. Casein, a protein

7. Can interfere with absorption of other minerals, especially copper, which gets crowded out of absorption sites. Anemia can result. High zinc intakes may also lower HDL-cholesterol (the "good" kind) in the blood.

8. High fluoride intakes cause a discoloration, or mottling, of the teeth. Some people believe there might be a cancer link to overdoses of fluoride.

9. Possibly only trace minerals may be low, but organic farming methods can put them back. Taking supplements on a regular basis can cause imbalances, as some may crowd out others in competing for the same absorption sites.

10. e

11. b

12. d

13. c

14. a

Practice Test: UNIT 13 — Vegan Foods I

ANSWER KEY

1. It is nutrients that are needed, not specific foods. All necessary nutrients can be gotten from plant-derived foods. It is meat (too much fat/protein, too little calcium) and dairy products (too much fat/protein, too little iron) that are "unbalanced."

2. Caloric density refers to the amount of calories in a food per given unit of weight or volume. Nutrient density refers to the amount of specific nutrients per calorie.

3. Citrus: oranges, grapefruits, lemons (good sources of C)
   Berries: strawberries, raspberries (good sources of C)
   Pomes: apples, pears (not much C)
   Stone fruits: peaches, apricots (not much C)
   Melons: honeydew, watermelon (good sources of C)

4. Potatoes are more like grains (ENB [CHO/Fat/Protein] = about 80/10/10). Avocados are high in fat (25/70/5). Most other vegetables average around 65/10/25.

5. Fruits average around 90/5/5, so they can be combined with vegetables in a diet to offset the slightly

high protein of the latter (25%).

6. Beta-carotene is a bright yellow-orange pigment. If a food is white or very pale in color it will be lacking. Other pigments, like chlorophyll, can mask the carotene, so vegetables like broccoli are good sources. Some foods, such as beets, have other pigments that provide color but are low in beta-carotene.

7. All animal products rank poorly in regard to environmental contamination because animals are higher in the food chain than plants; their flesh, milk, and eggs contain many times the concentration of pollutants. One of the factors that led to the banning of the use of the pesticide DDT in the United States several decades ago was a study that showed that the breast milk of women was exceeding the level allowable for public sale in cow's milk. The breast milk of human vegetarian women was analyzed and found to contain low DDT levels.

Practice Test: UNIT 14 — Vegan Foods II

ANSWER KEY

1. e

2. f

3. a

4. b

5. c

6. d

7. d

8. b

9. c

10. d

11. a

12. Much higher fat (42% of kcal vs. about 5% for most other beans) and slightly higher protein (37% of kcal vs. about 25%) content.

13. Both are soy products; tofu is made from soy milk and therefore has very little fiber. Tempeh is made from the whole bean, so it is rich in fiber. Tofu is often made with a calcium "salt," so it may be very rich in calcium.

14. Their ENB is more like nuts (except chestnuts) in that they are very high in fat.

15. They have hydrogenated fats added to prevent separation and prolong shelf life (after opening) without refrigeration. Natural peanut butter should be refrigerated to prevent rancidity.

16. Any oily substance in suspension in a watery substance.

17. Fiber present (if not strained)
    Lower fat, no cholesterol
    Lower sodium
    More moderate protein
    No lactose
    Less environmental contamination

18. Mashed tofu
    Arrowroot powder
    Dried apricots or flax seeds blended in water

19. 40; 140

Practice Test: UNIT 15 — Diet-Related Chronic Disease I

ANSWER KEY

1. *Acute deficiency disease*: Condition caused by lack of one or more essential nutrients; severe symptoms occur within a relatively short period of time.

   Chronic disease: Conditions that can be present for long periods of time before consequences become very serious. It is likely that their causes are chronic as well (diet, smoking, lack of exercise, etc.).

   Ischemia: Any situation in which blood flow is cut off to any tissue due to blockage or constriction of the supplying blood vessel.

   Myocardial infarction: Loss of functioning of heart muscle tissue, usually due to ischemia in that area.

   Atherosclerosis: Buildup of plaque in the larger or medium-sized blood vessels.

   Arteriosclerosis: Buildup of plaque in the smaller blood vessels.

   Coronary heart disease: Any disease involving the coronary blood flow, but most commonly caused by atherosclerotic plaque buildup.

Stroke: Loss of blood flow to the brain caused by rupture of a blood vessel leading to the brain, usually from plaque buildup.

Hypertension: Elevation in blood pressure; buildup of plaque can contribute to it (as vessels become smaller, the blood has to be pumped at a higher pressure to get it around the body). Hypertension is generally without symptoms.

2.   Switching to a vegan diet generally lowers one's blood pressure about 10 mm Hg. It has been theorized that the same stress hormones in meat extract that may cause superfluous stomach acid secretion might also cause blood pressure to rise. It is well known that stress increases blood pressure.

3.   When the heart gradually loses its capability for normal function (most frequently from complications of atherosclerosis), a set of bodily events occur that culminates in a condition in which the kidneys are unable to excrete sodium adequately. This results in fluid retention (water stays behind with the salt) known as edema. It is not caused by excess sodium, but sodium must be restricted while it is occurring.

4.   Initiators are what are usually called carcinogens, or those compounds capable of causing mutation in cells sufficient to bring about the change to a cancerous state. Promoters are those substances that encourage the growth of cancer cells once they have been formed.

5.   Fiber, cruciferous (cabbage family) vegetables, and the antioxidant nutrients: vitamins A (as beta-carotene only), C, E and the trace mineral selenium.

Practice Test: UNIT 16 — Diet-Related Chronic Disease II

ANSWER KEY

1.   Insulin-dependent (IDDM) and noninsulin-dependent (NIDDM) depending on whether the individual needs insulin to control blood glucose rise, or if it can be controlled through diet alone.

2.   Carbohydrates do not cause diabetes; controlling fat intake is a key, as is making sure CHO that is eaten is unrefined so that fiber helps regulate blood glucose rise.

3.   Fiber and fat content, as well as cooking time and method, are among other factors that seem to play a role in determining how the blood glucose rise will be affected.

4.   Cow's milk may be responsible for destroying the insulin-making mechanism in susceptible infants, thereby bringing on insulin-dependent diabetes mellitus.

5.   It was thought that the protein loss of nephrotic syndrome needed to be made up for; it is now realized that the less taken in, the less lost.

6.   Possibly because of lower cholesterol and phosphorus intake.

7. Excess protein
   Excess phosphorus
   Excess pre-formed Vitamin A and/or D
   Lack of exercise
   Cigarette smoking

8. Osteoarthritis
   Rheumatoid arthritis
   Gout

9. Used for detecting food allergies: consumption of only the least allergenic foods (rice, pears, carrots, etc.) for two weeks, then introduction of suspected allergens for a day or two each to see if symptoms reappear.

Practice Test: UNIT 17 — Life Cycle & Veganism

ANSWER KEY

1. Most nutrient needs are not doubled over the pre-pregnancy state; notably, calorie need is only about 15% higher. Thus, eating for two can lead to excess weight gain. Also many minerals are absorbed much better, so increased intake may not be necessary at all.

2. Folacin

3. Amounts of nutrients (protein, etc.) already appropriate
   Nutrients more easily absorbed
   Readily digestible (no need for heating)
   Immunity-granting antibodies
   Promotes growth of "friendly" microorganisms in infant's intestines

4. i.   cereals
   ii. vegetables
   iii. fruits
   iv. beans
   v.   nuts

5. For those who do grow more slowly, they "catch up" as they mature; there is the strong possibility that this later maturation is more ideal for avoiding certain diseases, especially cancers.

6. The amount needed per unit of ideal body weight declines with age.

7. Decrease in activity level, decrease in muscle mass, resulting in lower BMR; caloric intake remains constant (or may increase with increasing affluence).

8. Loss of teeth to bite and chew them, loss of strength and mobility for transporting these bulky items. Can be overcome with food processor, buying smaller quantities, sharing with others, etc.

9. Moderate exposure to sunlight, supplements, or a yearly injection are all effective.

Practice Test: UNIT 18 — Summary of Risks & Benefits of Vegan Diets

ANSWER KEY

1. *Calories*: Because of the higher fiber content of most vegan diets, there is a tendency to eat fewer calories if the same volume of food is eaten. This can easily be overcome (unless one wants to lose weight) by just eating a greater volume of food at each meal and/or by eating more frequent meals.

2. *Protein*: Probably the only legitimate worries about protein vegans should have is if they eat an all-fruit diet or if they feed very small children too much fiber, such that protein (and other nutrients) don't get absorbed adequately.

3. *Iron*: Vegetarians often replace high-iron meats with low-iron dairy products, sometimes resulting in iron-deficiency anemia. Obviously this can be overcome by reducing dairy consumption to a minimum or eliminating it altogether. Iron supplements are a less optimal option.

4. *Vitamin B-12*: Found only in animal products and in microorganism-rich supplemental foods (such as nutritional yeast), the prudent thing for vegans to do is to assure an occasional supply through fortified foods or supplements, though many vegans continue to live long, healthful, energetic lives without doing so.

5. See Answer Key to Practice Test 3 for formulae.

What would you say about the appropriateness of this balance?
Should be around 80% CHO, 10% Fat, 10% Protein

If not ideal, which food might you add more of to balance it better?
Whichever helps achieve the balance above.

How much would you add?
Varies according to extent of imbalance.

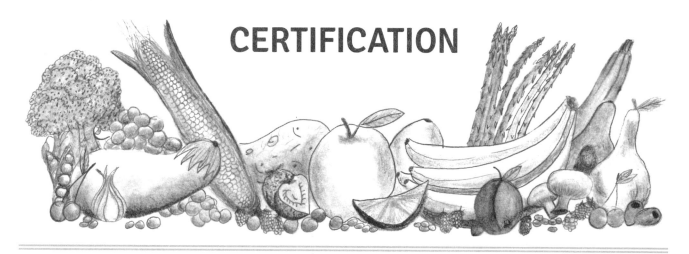

CERTIFICATION

Obtaining a Certificate for Completing This Course

Since this book is (as of this writing) identical to the material provided in the VEGEDINE Correspondence Course in Vegan Nutrition, you may elect to apply to receive a Certificate of Educational Achievement in Vegan Nutrition from The Association of Vegetarian Dietitians and Nutrition Educators (VEGEDINE). In order to earn the certificate you must take a series of three written tests, which are based almost entirely on the Practice Tests herein. These written tests must be proctored (witnessed) by an individual over the age of 18 who co-signs each test to the effect that it was taken within the prescribed time limit (two hours each) and without assistance of any kind. Your proctor must have a mailing address different than yours.

The current (2015) testing fee is $36 (US), and the Certificate Fee is $9, for a total of $45. Should the student fail to achieve a passing grade (average of 70% correct), the $9 Certificate Fee will be returned. To enroll, fill out the application below and send—along with the $45 testing and certificate fee payable to "VEGEDINE"—to the following address:

VEGEDINE Course
427 South Franklin Street
Watkins Glen, NY 14891

Vegetarian Dietitians and Nutrition Educators (VEGEDINE) Course in Vegan Nutrition
APPLICATION FOR TESTING-ONLY ENROLLMENT

Name:

Mailing Address:

Telephone: *Date of Birth:*

Last four digits of Social Security Number (or other ID number):

Name and address (address must be different than your own) of person who will proctor (witness) your tests:

Your Signature:

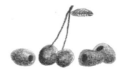

Appendix 1

Dr. Michael Greger's Recommendations for Optimum Vegan Nutrition

Michael Greger is a medical doctor specializing in vegan nutrition. He has gathered the following recommendations based on data gathered from studies of vegans and their typical food intakes. These recommendations would therefore help eliminate the common problems vegans encounter in seeking to avoid nutritional deficiencies. The information below is paraphrased from his website at http://www.veganMD.org.

Vitamin B-12

While needed in only tiny amounts, this nutrient can cause big problems if neglected too long. The more that is taken in at one time, the less percentage of it will be absorbed into the body, so: have twice-a-day (several hours apart) servings of B-12 fortified foods, each containing at least 20% of the recommended daily value of B-12. Examples are a cup of fortified soy or fortified rice milk, or a teaspoon of vegetarian-support formula nutritional yeast. The daily value of B-12 is 6 micrograms (mcg). Thus, 20% of 6 = 1.2 mcg, twice daily = 2.4 mcg, which is an adequate amount if consumed in this manner. If daily supplements are chosen instead, take at least 10 mcg. Tablets should be chewed or dissolved under tongue for ideal absorption. A weekly supplement is a third option: take one 2,000 mcg tablet (chew or dissolve under tongue) once a week.

Essential Fatty Acids

To ensure adequate omega-3 intake, consume two tablespoons of ground flax seeds daily. In addition, avoid anything with "partially hydrogenated" on the ingredient label. Also avoid deep-fried foods, and limit oils rich in omega-6 (corn, cottonseed, safflower, sunflower). Pregnant or breastfeeding women and people with diabetes may not be able to convert the alpha-linolenic acid to DHA adequately, so should seek to consume 300 mg of DHA (there are plant sources) daily.

Vitamin D

If you can't get adequate sunshine, ensure an intake of 400 international units (IU) daily by eating mushrooms, using fortified cereals, juices, milks, and/or taking supplements. Common white mushrooms have 70 IU in one cup; other types (chanterelle, shiitake) have considerably higher amounts.

Calcium

If you can't consume lots of leafy greens (don't count on high-oxalate ones like spinach, chard, and beet greens, though), try to get 700–1,000 mg each day from fortified foods and/or supplements.

Iodine

Try to get about 75 mcg daily (or twice that 3 times a week) from seaweed, iodized salt, and/or supplements.

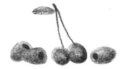

Appendix 1

Dr. Michael Greger's Recommendations for Optimum Vegan Nutrition

Iron
Combine iron-rich and vitamin C-rich foods at meals.

Selenium
Eating about 20 Brazil nuts each month ensures an adequate intake if you happen to live in (or eat from) an area with selenium-poor soils, such as northern Europe.

Drink at least five cups of water a day. Eat dark leafy greens, beans, nuts, fresh fruits, and whole grains every day. Eat as many vegetables as you can...at least a pound a day.

Appendix 2

Breast Cancer, Prostate Cancer & Consumption of Animal Foods

The following quotes, compiled from the books Eat to Live *by Joel Fuhrman, MD,* The China Study *by T. Colin Campbell, and* Your Life in Your Hands *by Jane A. Plant, suggest the similarity between these serious common hormone-related cancers and their powerful link to consumption of animal products, especially dairy foods.*

—Men with a family history of breast cancer have an increased risk of prostate cancer, and women with a family history of prostate cancer have an increased risk of breast cancer. *Epidemiology* 9 (5) (1998) 525–529.

—There is a link between animal protein and cancer, evident in both laboratory and human epidemiological studies. *Journal of Surgical Research* 59 (2) (1995) 225–228.

—A massive international study that contained data from 59 countries showed that men who ate the most meat, poultry, and dairy products were the most likely to die from prostate cancer, while those who ate the most unrefined plant foods were the least likely to die from this disease. *Journal of the National Cancer Institute* 90 (21) (1998) 1637–1647.

—As animal-derived food intake increases from once a week to four times a week, breast cancer rates increase by 70%. *Japanese Journal of Cancer Research* 85 (1994) 572–577.

—A British study found low death rates for breast cancer where dairy product consumption was low, even when intake of other fats was high. *British Journal of Cancer* 24 (1970), 633–43.

—Studies that have failed to show a relationship between animal product consumption and breast cancer suffer from methodological problems. *Journal of the National Cancer Institute* 89 (1997) 766–775. *Note: Insulin-like Growth Factor-1 (IGF-1) is a growth hormone produced by all mammals. Levels of it are very high in dairy products and in beef products made from the flesh of dairy cows, since these animals are bred to grow very quickly and to produce a lot of milk so their calves can grow quickly.*

—In a study of 700 men, 233 of whom were vegan, serum IGF-1 was 9% lower in the vegans. *British Journal of Cancer* 83(1) (2000) 95–97.

—In a study of men with prostate cancer, it was found that on average their serum IGF-1 was 8% higher than matched controls without active prostate cancer. *Science* 279 (1998), 563–6.

Appendix 2

Breast Cancer, Prostate Cancer & Consumption of Animal Foods

Thus, a vegan diet lowers IGF-1 by 9%, a seemingly minor amount, yet an 8% difference is all that is seen between healthy and cancer-ridden individuals. IGF-1 is apparently a powerful hormone that only needs a slight elevation above normal to cause damage.

—Among women younger than 50, having high IGF-1 levels raises breast cancer risk by seven times. *Lancet* 351 (1998), 1393–96.

—The 1,25 form of vitamin D in the body is lowered by diets rich in animal protein and/or too high in calcium. When blood levels of 1,25 vitamin D are depressed, IGF-1 becomes more active. Together these factors increase the birth of new cells while simultaneously inhibiting the removal of old cells, both favoring the development of cancer. This can result in 9.5 times increased risk of advanced stage prostate cancer. *Journal of National Cancer Institute* 94 (2002) 1099–1109.

—Undoubtedly, the best anticancer diet would be completely vegan: strictly vegetarian, with no meat or dairy products. *Your Life in Your Hands, Understanding, Preventing and Overcoming Breast Cancer* by Dr. Jane A. Plant, pg. 122.

And finally…in case there is still worry that a dairy-free diet can lead to osteoporosis:

—The Nurses' Health Study (over 120,000 subjects) found that the consumption of milk does not protect against hip or forearm fractures. Those who drank three or more servings of milk a day actually had a slightly higher rate of fractures than women who drank little or no milk. *American Journal of Public Health* 87 (1997) 992–997.

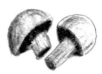

Appendix 3

Dairy Products & Ovarian Cancer Risk

A study published in the *American Journal of Clinical Nutrition* (Vol. 80, No. 5, 1353-1357, November 2004), which followed over 60,000 women for 13 years, found that drinking more than two glasses of milk a day significantly upped the risk of the most serious form of ovarian cancer. Dairy products had previously been linked to cancers, including those of the breast and prostate. The researchers found women who consumed more than four servings of dairy products a day had twice the risk of serous ovarian cancer than women who had fewer than two. They found that milk had the strongest link with ovarian cancer; those women who drank two or more glasses a day were at double the risk of those who did not consume it at all or only in small amounts. The reason why milk may increase the risk of ovarian cancer is unclear, but one theory is that lactose, a type of sugar found in milk, might over stimulate production of hormones, which encourage tumor growth.

In an article entitled "A Prospective Study of Dietary Lactose and Ovarian Cancer" in the *International Journal of Cancer* (10 June 2004; 110 (2): 271-7), authors K.M. Fairfield *et al* of the Department of Medicine, Brigham and Women's Hospital, Harvard Medical School, studied lactose, milk, and milk product consumption in relation to ovarian cancer risk among over 80,000 nurses from 1976 to 1996. They observed a twofold higher risk of the serous ovarian cancer subtype (the most common and most deadly form of the disease) among those in the highest category of lactose consumption compared to the lowest (RR 2.07, 95% CI, 1.27–3.40). For each 11 gram increase in lactose consumption (the approximate amount in one glass of milk), they observed a 20% increase in risk of serous cancers (RR 1.20, 95% CI, 1.04–1.39). Skim and low-fat milk were the largest contributors to dietary lactose. Women who consumed one or more servings of skim or low-fat milk daily had a 32% higher risk of any ovarian cancer (RR 1.32, 95% CI, 0.97–1.82) and a 69% higher risk of serous ovarian cancer (RR 1.69, 95% CI, 1.12–2.56) compared to women consuming three or less servings monthly. Controlling for fat intake did not change their findings.

As far back as 1989, a study done by researchers at Harvard University suggested that women who ate the most dairy products, especially yogurt, were much more likely to develop ovarian cancer (*Lancet* 2, 66-71).

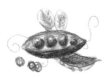

Index

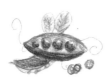

Index

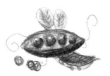

Index